Liberation

–

The Fruition of Yoga

Yogani

From The AYP Enlightenment Series

AYP Publishing

For ordering information go to:

www.advancedyogapractices.com

Published simultaneously in:

Nashville, Tennessee, U.S.A.
London, England, U.K.
Melbourne, Australia

ISBN 978-1-938594-00-7 (Paperback)
ISBN 978-1-938594-01-4 (eBook)

In the modern era,
Everyone can sample liberation for a short while.
What we do after that will make all the difference.

iv – Liberation

Introduction

This concise volume provides a survey of the methods of Yoga as they relate to the rise of the *non-dual* condition of enlightenment, or *Liberation* (*Moksha* in Sanskrit), and practices that can be utilized during the end stage of the journey. It is about the rise of the *witness* and the evolution to *ripeness* and *relational self-inquiry* for permanent realization of the observer being both beyond and in *unity* with all objects of perception, accompanied by the natural emergence of an unending flow of divine love in the world.

While this book is about *Advaita-Vedanta* and *Jnana Yoga* for end stage realization, it is also about assuring that the prerequisites of *Deep Meditation* and related yogic methods are not ignored, as so often happens in modern teachings on enlightenment.

Liberation is the cap-stone of the *AYP Enlightenment Series*, the *vedanta* of it so to speak, meaning, "the end of knowledge." It is also an expansion on the discussion that began in the seventh book of the series: *Self-Inquiry*. As we have always said, the center of all spiritual progress is found within each human being, and that theme culminates here. Liberation is in your hands.

The AYP Enlightenment Series has been an endeavor to present the most effective methods of spiritual practice in a series of easy-to-read books that anyone can use to gain practical results immediately and over the long term. For centuries, many of these powerful practices have been shrouded in secrecy, mainly in an effort to preserve them. Now we find ourselves in the *information age*, and able to preserve knowledge for present and future generations like never before. The question remains: "How far can we go in effectively transmitting spiritual methods in writing?"

Since the beginning in 2003, the writings of AYP have been an experiment to see just how much can be conveyed, with much more detail included on practices than in the spiritual writings of the past. Can books provide us the specific means necessary to tread the path to enlightenment, or do we have to surrender at the feet of a *guru* to find our salvation? Well, clearly we must surrender to something, even if it is to our own innate potential to live a freer and happier life. If we are able to do that, and maintain regular practice, then books like this one can come alive and instruct us in the ways of human spiritual transformation. If the reader is ready and the book is worthy, amazing things can happen.

While one person's name is given as the author of this book, it is actually a distillation of the efforts of thousands of practitioners over thousands of years. This is one person's attempt to simplify and make practical the spiritual methods that many have demonstrated throughout history. All who have gone before have my deepest gratitude, as do the many I am privileged to be in touch with in the present who continue to practice with dedication and good results.

I hope you will find this book to be a useful resource as you travel along your chosen path.

Practice wisely, and enjoy!

Table of Contents

Chapter 1 – A Path from Here to Here

We live in an amazing time, one when access to the tools of enlightenment is becoming increasingly available due to vastly improved worldwide communications. The causes and effects of human spiritual transformation are being revealed by science, and are being experienced first-hand by countless practitioners around the world. The obstacles to clear seeing are many and it is not an easy task to find our way through them all. Nevertheless, the task has been undertaken, and the relentless rise of human consciousness everywhere cannot be denied.

What many are realizing is that spiritual enlightenment, also called *liberation* (or *moksha* in Sanskrit), is here and now, in this place and in this moment. This is why, after years or decades of traveling a spiritual path, the ones who have gone the distance may well exclaim, "The path leads from here to here!"

The logic of this is very simple: The world we see reflected in our mind via the senses is a creation of our own identification with the objects of our perception, beginning with our sense of self, our sense of "*I*" as an entity that is real with rights of ownership in this world. But is it real, and does it have rights of ownership?

Think about it. What do you own? Who is there to own anything? The experience of "*I*," the feeling of it, is a conditioned response that we have been living with since early childhood. The only reason it remains is because we have not yet evolved to a sense of self that is beyond the realm of time and space, the realm where we believe we can own things. Yes, custodians we are. Owners? Impossible. If we did own this realm, we would not have to leave it, and we all do. At most, we are borrowing this realm for a short time, and then we are out of here. Of course there are many ways we try to get around our limited stay here, by making a big name, a big fortune, or a big impact on humanity, so that we will be remembered. But what difference will it make to us? None. Zilch. At best we are providing a service of unselfish giving so others who come after us may have an easier time of it here. At worst, we may harm millions and be vilified for the rest of human history. Those are the extremes. Most of us fall somewhere in-between. None of it makes much difference in the long run.

But something matters. We can feel it in our bones. Nature is always evolving toward a more perfect expression, never quite getting there, but never giving up either. That impulse lives in us also, the unceasing flow toward becoming more. It does not only apply to our activities on this earth, but also to revealing our inner nature in this life. Intuitively, we know there is immortality within us, something that transcends all that comes and goes here, and our tendency to get tangled up in it.

There is such a thing as *liberation*, and that is what we'd like to explore in this book, particularly as it relates to the ancient and ever-new field of *yoga*.

When we combine the ancient wisdom with modern ways of applying and disseminating the knowledge, we begin to see the journey of human spiritual transformation in ways that were not even imaginable a few decades ago. In doing so, we will be stepping across imaginary lines of demarcation, shedding centuries of sectarian confusion, including some of it that is still with us today, but fading rapidly in the light of knowledge and direct experience.

Is Instant Enlightenment Possible?

Anything is possible on the spiritual path. However, to regard instant enlightenment, a simple mental realization, as a reality for everyone is simply unrealistic. If it were so, the world would be radically different than it is today.

There is a teaching out there that we can see the truth in the here and now, and that all the other things we may have been doing, or are considering doing for our spiritual betterment have been and are a complete waste of time. We often hear this from teachers who have spent decades in meditation and other spiritual practices, who one day had the *Aha* that marked their awakening into liberation, and then said, "Why did I waste so many years in practices, when I could have woken up way back then?" They advise that we should just let go now, and it will happen, just as it did for them (after countless meditation sittings over many years).

Enlightened people seem to have short memories. Can we actually wish ourselves from New York to California without making the journey?

The truth is, an awakening is always "instant," an *Aha* we have seen in all the awakenings experienced up until now, and in all the awakenings that are sure to come after. While such epiphanies (openings) may seem instant and can be very profound, we tend to categorize them as self-sufficient final events, which they are not. We tend to uncouple effects from their causes. It is a normal oversight, forgetting what we did yesterday that set the stage for what we are doing today. However, in spiritual matters, the forgetting is not a help to others, or even to ourselves as we make false assumptions about our spiritual condition (more on that later).

What got us to past awakenings, and will surely get us to all future ones, is spiritual practice of one kind or other. While the fruit of our labor is good, how the fruit came to be is of far greater importance to those of us who would like to harvest more fruit for ourselves, and help others do the same.

So, while enlightenment is always hiding in plain sight, coming into a permanent direct realization of it is a process.

Suppose we have a big awakening on the front end, such as, "Oh my goodness, there is no 'me,' only this unending unfoldment of life."

Even with this, there will be much more work to do. Many in this modern age are having this kind of experience, a *sampling* of liberation. It is like a temporary clearing of the clouds, revealing the radiant sunshine. But then the clouds come back in and we don't see it fully anymore. Experiences like this provide a powerful inspiration that can carry us forward on our path for a long time. While we likely can't will the clouds to part again right away, there is much we can do in a systematic way to gradually dissolve them, which bit-by-bit makes the clouds thinner and increasingly wispy. Then our seeing gradually becomes more and more, until one day we are bathed in the full sunlight 24 hours per day, 7 days per week. So our initial opening and the inspiration it provides, if followed up on wisely, can bring us into full realization. What we do between the initial inspiration and the end stage will make all the difference. Systematic practice is the surest path, assuming we approach it with prudence, and avoid the mental traps along the way. We will talk about the pitfalls and blind alleys later in this book. They are all too common.

But first, let's develop a baseline of knowledge about what it takes to move steadily forward toward liberation. In doing so, we can assure our continued progress and move beyond the unrealistic expectations and imaginings that can delay us on our path.

A Process of Purification and Opening

There are many ways to look at the process of human spiritual transformation – everything from overcoming/destroying the ego to cleaning the inner windows of perception. No matter how we look at it, it is the same process – a journey, a path, or some sort of undertaking leading from an unrealized state to a realized state. In the end we find that we have gone from here to here, from seeing the world inaccurately as division and limitation to seeing it truly for what it is as *unity* and infinite expression, and experiencing the profound freedom that comes with that awakening. As it says in the Bible:

"You will know the truth and the truth will set you free."

There is no place to go. It is only our perception of life here and now that will change. This can have a profound impact on our conduct in the world, but on the surface we will still seem quite the ordinary person we were before. Perhaps even more ordinary, because we will be more fulfilled in the moment.

As the Zen Buddhists say: "Before enlightenment, chop wood, carry water. After enlightenment, chop wood, carry water."

From the point of view of yoga, the path is one of purification and opening. We mean this on every level from the gross physical to the finest strata of our neurobiology, mind, emotions, and beyond into the realm of the pure consciousness underlying all of existence. The methods of yoga are for undertaking this global process of purification and opening. We could even say it is a cosmic undertaking, because at the deepest level of our nature, we are one and the same as the entire cosmos. Every human being is like a hologram, able to reflect the infinite in this earth realm.

When we say "purification," what do we mean? If we consider the cloud analogy again, we can see that the clouds block our view of the sun, except when they part temporarily, which may be a somewhat random event. They will no longer block the sun at all if they can be permanently dissolved by systematic means, which is not random. It is cause and effect. This dissolving of obstructions (the clouds) to clear our vision is the purification we are talking about. Likewise, obstructions embedded deep in our nervous system can block clear vision of the true nature of ourselves and of all life.

Looking at it another way, our perception is much like looking through the windshield of a car. If the windshield is dirty, we will not see much, and our driving will be erratic and hazardous. When the windshield has been cleaned, our vision will be clear and our driving will be much better informed. So it is with our nervous system and our perception of the world. The purpose of the methods of yoga is to clean the windshield of our perception, this vehicle of our conscious life, which has the ability to be opened literally to the infinite. That is what we are, the infinite expressing through this limited form in time and space. Realization, or enlightenment, is the ongoing direct experience of the unlimited nature of ourselves. So this windshield cleaning thing that we call *yoga* is a high stakes game. It is the joining of our unlimited inner nature with our limited outer nature, and its implications are profound.

As we systematically apply the methods of yoga on a daily basis over time, the resulting inner purification and opening will be experienced in a variety of ways. We may have symptoms of purification, which can range from profound and ecstatic to dull, or downright uncomfortable. There are means provided for stabilizing the extremes of experience, so we can continue on our way with minimum disruption or delay. But, primarily, we will notice a gradual unfoldment characterized by rising abiding inner silence, ecstatic bliss and an outpouring of divine love through us leading to an experience of *unity* and freedom in this life.

The rise of *abiding inner silence* has been called *witnessing*, meaning that initially we come to view all objects of perception as being outside our shifting sense of self, which is untouched by external events in the realm of stillness. This sense of witnessing is none other than the rise of abiding inner silence within us. This separation dissolves later, as we move beyond witnessing into a non-dual condition where our sense of self becomes unified, encompassing all that is. Interestingly, this expansion of self corresponds to the loss of the binding influence of the sense of "*I, me, and mine*" as our identity, though we may act in the world much as we did before. As mentioned earlier, nothing really changes except our perception.

On the ecstatic side of it (what we sometimes refer to as the energetic side, or *Kundalini*), there is an awakening that is centered in the spinal nerve, expanding gradually outward from there.

There is a relationship between inner silence and the rise of ecstasy that leads to a *marriage* of these two awakening spiritual components within us. This marriage is for the purpose of enabling inner silence to move in the world. We have called it "*stillness in action*." In fact, the relationship between inner silence and ecstasy forms the perceptual structure for our life to become an ongoing divine outpouring, which is also the process of "*I, me, and mine*" merging into *unity*.

What is the end result of all this? Freedom in this life. At the same time, as we undergo this process, we are also becoming an increasing influence in visible and invisible ways for others to unfold freedom in their lives.

So this path of purification and opening is well worth undertaking. By helping ourselves become free, we are helping everyone become free. It is one of the greatest benefits of our liberation. We can do it for ourselves, but as the clouds clear, we come to realize that we are doing it for everyone. When the sun is shining brightly, it warms everyone.

It is a nice scenario, and perhaps it sounds a bit idealistic and theoretical. It surely would be only that, if we could not provide effective means for making the journey from here to here.

So let's look at the means.

Chapter 2 – Ways and Means

There are innumerable ways to approach the process of human spiritual transformation. Even within the field of yoga, there are many approaches, ranging from focusing almost exclusively on physical practices, to focusing almost exclusively on mental practices. Paths that are primarily devotional are yoga also. The most effective approaches, whether called "yoga" or not, will include elements from all three of these aspects of our nature: body, mind and emotion.

Whatever the approach may be, all effective spiritual practice originates within the human being. With the methods of yoga, we are stimulating inherent abilities we have to evolve as vehicles, or channels, of pure bliss consciousness in the world.

In traditional approaches to spiritual development, we are often told that the teachings and techniques we use define our spirituality. It is just the opposite. It is our inner tendencies and abilities that determine the ways and means that can be applied to accelerate our purification and opening. All of the spiritual traditions of the world have their origin within human beings. Human beings are the source of pure knowledge coming from beyond, and also the source of the many distortions that occur due to the obstructions that exist within us. So, in a very real sense, all spiritual methods and traditions are *bootstrapping* operations, where we are harvesting pure knowledge (hopefully) from a sea of muddy water. As our inner clarity improves over time, as our windshield becomes cleaner, we are much better able to separate the clear water from the mud. So progress tends to accelerate the further we go, as does the quality of our inner and outer life.

When offered in an open, well-integrated format, like we do at AYP, the tools of yoga offer the opportunity for flexible application on the journey, according to individual need. With such a resource, we can focus on developing the primary components of enlightenment: the cultivation of abiding inner silence and ecstatic conductivity in the human nervous system, which, blended together, enable awareness to evolve beyond the limitations and suffering associated with excessive identification with "*I, me, and mine.*"

Yoga Practices

Many have the impression that yoga is about postures, with maybe some breathing exercises (pranayama) added. When meditation is considered, that is often viewed to be something outside the mainstream of yoga. And when it comes to self-inquiry methods, the domain of *advaita-vedanta* (non-duality), it isn't considered to be yoga at all.

It turns out none of these assessments are correct. Not only does yoga include full scope practices such as asanas (postures), pranayama (breathing techniques), deep meditation and additional methods, it also includes special measures (like samyama) that lead to and support non-dual self-inquiry – *Jnana Yoga*, which means union through direct knowledge.

So what is missing from yoga? Not much. In fact, the eight limbs of yoga, postulated by Patanjali centuries ago, form a good checklist for assessing any path of spiritual practice for completeness.

As mentioned, it is the human nervous system that determines the process of spiritual unfoldment, and yoga covers every aspect.

Here is a review of the Eight Limbs of Yoga:

- **Yama** (*restraints* – non-violence, truthfulness, non-stealing, preservation and cultivation of sexual energy, and non-covetousness)
- **Niyama** (*observances* – purity, contentment, spiritual intensity, study of spiritual knowledge and *Self*, and active surrender to the divine)
- **Asana** (postures and physical maneuvers)
- **Pranayama** (breathing techniques)
- **Pratyahara** (introversion of the senses)
- **Dharana** (systematic attention on an object)
- **Dhyana** (meditation – systematic dissolving of the object in consciousness)
- **Samadhi** (absorption in pure bliss consciousness)

And there is that special additional category of practice called **Samyama,** which employs the last three limbs of yoga simultaneously in reverse order, bringing *stillness* out to penetrate all of our thinking, feeling and daily activity. It is a very important practice for cultivating *ripeness* and end stage enlightenment.

Traditionally, the eight limbs of yoga have been taught in order. But in modern times we have seen variations in the order to optimize the evolution of human spiritual tendencies for purification and opening. In the AYP approach we begin with spiritual desire (*bhakti*) and go straight to deep meditation (*dharana* and *dhyana*), which cultivates abiding inner silence (*samadhi*). Then spinal breathing pranayama, asanas, mudras, bandhas and tantric methods are added according individual preference to facilitate the process of awakening ecstatic conductivity and radiance. Along the way, *samyama* is added to begin moving inner silence outward into the nervous system and the external environment in an increasing flow, which leads to increasing spiritual desire, and a natural tendency toward self-inquiry (*jnana*), service (karma yoga), and liberation (*moksha*).

Detailed instructions on all of the practices mentioned here (and more) are provided throughout the AYP writings. Our main focus in this book is on end stage development. Make sure to cover previous instructional writings in the *AYP Enlightenment Series*, beginning with *deep meditation* so you can take maximum advantage of the information in this volume.

The cultivation and movement of inner silence create the foundation for effective (relational) non-dual self-inquiry, the process of assimilating the witness state of consciousness and moving beyond it, dissolving subject-object identification, which leads to unending joyous freedom while remaining fully functional in this life.

We will go into more detail on this progression later in the book. While in the AYP approach we begin with deep meditation, this is not to say anyone cannot start anywhere in yoga practices Many begin with asanas these days, or even with self-inquiry only, and can find some progress. Of course, progress is a relative thing, and is it difficult to evaluate anyone's spiritual condition with certainty. In fact, claims of progress with various spiritual approaches may often be premature, if not exaggerations – building mental castles in the air, you know. It is very easy to do without even knowing it.

In the AYP approach, we avoid making such claims and comparisons, and rely primarily on the experience of each individual practitioner instead. What anyone's condition may be is unique to that person, and any measuring should be in relation to each practitioner's experience the day, month or year before. In other words, each person's journey to enlightenment is a continuum, and relevant only to their own directly experienced progress. We do provide general descriptions of various experiential milestones along the way, so anyone can see how they are doing, without getting too hung up on making comparisons with other practitioners. In this way, we endeavor to stick with the facts, rather than finding ourselves living in the flood of excessive claims that are so common in the aspiring world of human spiritual endeavor.

So it is a good idea to minimize proclamations and premature claims, especially to ourselves. If we are feeling some peace, creativity and energy in daily life, that is good, and we can let it happen and progress naturally without a lot of fanfare.

When we start out, whether we begin with an inspiration coming from a non-dual epiphany, any other dramatic experience, or from a simple desire to improve our life, we will be embarking on a journey of practices. How we handle that will make all the difference in where we end up years later.

So let us practice wisely, and enjoy the fruit.

Symptoms of Human Spiritual Transformation

As mentioned in the previous section, the process of human spiritual transformation involves the cultivation of abiding inner silence, ecstatic energy, and a merging of these two, leading to a non-dual *unity* state. What are the symptoms of this unfoldment? Here are the key experiential characteristics:

- **Rise of Abiding Inner Silence** – Experienced as a sense of centeredness, *witnessing* of daily activity and sleep states as occurring outside immoveable silent self, more spontaneous energy and creativity, and less susceptibility to stress in everyday living.

- **Rise of Ecstatic Awakening** – Experienced as physical and emotional sensations of inner energy flow, the introversion and refinement of sensory perception, noticing of *ecstatic conductivity* in the body and *ecstatic radiance* beyond the body.

- **Rise of Unity** – Experience of merging of inner silence and ecstatic energy, manifesting as a natural *divine flow* coming from within during daily activity, and a sense of *ripening* in inquiry and more spontaneity of positive actions in the world. We come to know ourselves as *stillness in action*, beyond our prior sense of "*I, me, and mine,*" and beyond the subject/object duality of earlier stages of *witnessing*.

Much can be said about these experiential stages. First, it should be emphasized that each category of experience corresponds with undertaking particular practices on a daily basis over the long term. With an effective integration of practices, paced to suit our individual tendencies and inclinations, a balanced unfoldment can be achieved.

The rise of abiding inner silence (*witness*) results mainly from daily deep meditation, and is by far the most revealing and practical of symptoms on the way to enlightenment. We could even say that the rise of abiding inner silence is the only benefit that counts, because from that, all the rest will flow automatically.

We may first notice abiding inner silence as a peaceful sense of separation from the ups and downs of life. Later on, or perhaps when we experience a sudden event like an accident or sudden noise, we will notice that we *witness* events in a way that is untouched, leaving much less of an impression in our awareness and nervous system. It will be a new experience, and we will get used to it as our normal way of being. It is a sense of freedom creeping up on us, which can happen even in the early days of our meditation. It accumulates over time, and takes on increasingly broad dimensions.

There can be some energy flowing within us (second category of symptoms) from deep meditation alone. With the addition of spinal breathing pranayama, asanas, mudras, bandhas, and tantric methods, the expansion of ecstatic conductivity will become much more pronounced, as a current between our root (perineum) and brow (third eye). It may begin as a very thin current, corresponding to our spinal nerve (sushumna), and over time expand from that center thread to encompass our whole body, and beyond, with ecstatic radiance. Along with that, we may experience visions, sounds and sensations in our expanding interior, which may be found to be occurring simultaneously both inside and outside our body, a sensory paradox. This is the introversion of sensory experience.

The energetic stage of opening, also called *kundalini*, can be quite dramatic and sometimes distracting. It will be good to remind ourselves that experiences are not the cause of spiritual progress. Practices are. Having a good amount of abiding inner silence (witness quality) cultivated before we pursue an energetic awakening will be a big plus, enabling us to take the potentially dramatic experiences in stride. In time, the energetic experiences will settle down and become blended with abiding inner silence. At this time, we will begin to feel our life and the events around us occurring increasingly as a *flow in stillness*. We could even say a *divine flow*, because life takes on that sort of uplifting celestial quality. We find that we are the stillness behind it all, and also doing the action in our daily life in an elevated way. We can then know the paradox of our life being *stillness in action*. It is the beginning of liberation.

None of this is to say there will not be some bumps along the way. Difficulties can occur, especially on the energetic side of the enlightenment equation, which can result from overdoing with any of the practices mentioned so far. Sometimes the energy flow will be more than the purifying and opening nervous system can easily accommodate. A sense of being stuck, or even physical and/or emotional discomfort can occur. These excesses are sometimes referred to as *kundalini symptoms* and are clear signs that *self-pacing* of practices is necessary, plus engagement in activities that will aid us in the *grounding* and *integration* of the surging spiritual energies in the body and surroundings.

Such symptoms of excess can become quite uncomfortable if the practitioner assumes that breaking through is the way to go (it isn't), and puts too much emphasis on cultivating energetic symptoms directly, or if practices are inadvertently overdone without an understanding of the consequences, which can often be delayed in time. Hence, prudence is always in order when undertaking powerful spiritual practices. Less will often be more.

Due to the tendencies many of us may have toward overdoing, a key focus in the AYP writings is on keeping a healthy balance of practices for achieving maximum progress with comfort and safety. While it is not the purpose of this small book on end stage development to delve into all the measures utilized, it should be mentioned that there is extensive support available for those having difficulty with inner energies in the AYP writings and in the online support community. It should also be mentioned that while situations where energy experiences are getting out of hand when utilizing the AYP system are rare, it is fairly common to see practitioners coming from elsewhere with energy imbalances requiring assistance. Either way, there are extensive measures available within the AYP system for dealing with energy mishaps that may occur along the way.

Once the abiding inner silence and energy awakening stages are well underway, and blending together in our daily activity, we will notice a new way of looking at the world and ourselves arising in our life. We have already mentioned the merging of stillness with ecstatic energy, the resulting divine outpouring, stillness in action, and *unity*, but more will be necessary in the way of practices to accommodate these end stage developments.

Structured samyama practice is particularly important, because it sets the stage for our life becoming more and more lived from *within stillness*. This, in turn, facilitates self-inquiry and a gradually increasing divine flow in our life, with more inclination toward service, which then leads us into the *unity* experience. By then, it can barely be called an experience. The flow in *unity* is what we become, what we are.

Indeed, the whole idea of *experience* gets swallowed up in the dissolving of the subject, object, and mechanics of perceptual identification we have bought into since childhood. In the end stage of our journey, we become the whole thing, without identification. Then subject and objects (experiences) are seen to be passing like waves on the ocean of our being. We will see objective events within and around us, much the way we might see our internal blood flow now – automatic and functioning very well on its own accord. As we become less identified with "*I, me, and mine*," we see the truth and become free.

We each may come to this monumental transformation from a slightly different angle, which is why we do not insist on a fixed approach to practices, self-inquiry and end stage awakening. But the basic components of experience are going to be there regardless, no matter which approach we are using.

If one begins on their journey with self-inquiry only and finds a taste of *unity*, surely the abiding inner silence and energetic stages are going to be dealt with as well. Without a systematic approach it can get pretty messy. It is the basic mechanics of the neurobiology associated with human spiritual transformation. It is not occurring only in the mind.

Wherever the mind goes, so too must the body go, and vise versa. This is why those who pursue a stand-alone self-inquiry path often run into trouble. The purification and opening must occur on all levels, not only in the mind. The change goes deep into the subtle strata of the human being, to the level of our cells and DNA. Spiritual practices run that deep, and beyond.

This is why we talk so much about taking care of the prerequisites for enlightenment with deep meditation, spinal breathing pranayama, the physical practices, samyama and so on, before we place much emphasis on self-inquiry and other end stage practices. Once we have taken care of the prerequisites, it becomes a very different ball game. Then it all comes together in stillness. Even excessive *kundalini symptoms* can be quelled in relational self-inquiry.

This is what we mean by becoming *ripe*. Ripe for what? Ripe for liberation, of course!

On Becoming Ripe

In the terminology we have been using in AYP, "*ripe*" means "*relational*," which is the increasing presence of abiding inner silence (the *witness*), blending *in relationship* with all aspects of our daily life, including our self-inquiry into who or what we are. Before this, our thinking, feeling and action will be something like unripe fruit, missing that liberated fullness and radiant inner sweetness that is known when we experience ourselves to be the doer who is beyond all manifestations of doing in the realm of time and space.

We know when a piece of fruit is ripe, often just by looking at it or by its sweet scent, and surely when we bite into it. Likewise, those who are knowledgeable and would teach us the way of *advaita-vedanta* (non-duality and self-inquiry) will be able to tell whether we are ripe for it or not, and will interact with us accordingly. At least they should be able to. It is an essential distinction, not only for advancing our spiritual progress, but also for our wellbeing in everyday living.

If we are ripe, the methods of self-inquiry will be able to help us a lot. And if we are not ripe, the wisest course will be to engage in deep meditation and other practices that will bring us steadily into ripeness leading to *unity*.

Teachers who offer uncompromising approaches to *unity* via the immediate destruction of ego may do more harm than good if their methods are forced prematurely on the unripe aspirant. More importantly, the aspirant will either tolerate such teachers and teachings or not, according to their inner condition. In other words, there is only so much a non-duality teaching can accomplish until the time of ripeness has arrived. Once ripeness has arrived, those who teach non-duality can serve as *harvesters of enlightenment*, the *fruit pickers*. They will keep telling us the same thing: "You are *That* which is beyond all this." But if we are not ripe, we will not be able to hear it deep within.

Beyond some inner energetic nudging, few non-duality teachers are able to give practical means enabling us to become ripe for enlightenment. It is only in ripeness that we can fully absorb what they are saying and experience it directly in our own life. Becoming ripe is up to us, and we will likely have to look at a wider integrated routine of practices for assistance in that. That is just how it is.

On one hand, becoming ripe is something that will happen in its own course, depending on the practices for cultivation we are employing, or the lack of them. An orchard that is left on its own may become irregular and full of weeds. It may still produce some ripe fruit, but it will be an affair left much to chance. There are many random events that can happen to disrupt an orchard that is left untended. Whatever its inherent shortcomings may be will be left unaddressed.

On the other hand, the orchard that is well tended, cultivated and fertilized will yield ripe fruit with predictability – sweet luscious fruit that is ready to pick. It is very easy, because the cultivating is already done, and the fruit is ready to fall off the tree. Even without any special picking skills, the ripe fruit will fall off the tree, won't it?

Teachings that are genuine will be the first to advise a ripe aspirant, "You don't need these methods of self-inquiry. Just abide in who you are through thick and thin, knowing yourself to be the *One* behind all this, and you will see first hand the truth of life." This is living naturally beyond the imaginary dream realm of "*I, me, and mine.*"

Since the last half of the 20th century a lot has changed. Due to the increasingly widespread availability of effective spiritual practices, many more aspirants are becoming ripe than in centuries past, and the non-duality fruit picking has become much easier.

But let us not mistake the fruit picking with the process of good cultivation to ripeness. The fruit that is falling off the trees today has not been caused primarily by the fruit pickers. It has been caused by the millions around the world who have been cultivating abiding inner silence within themselves with meditation and related practices for decades.

Those who have taken responsibility for their spiritual cultivation are the ones who are bringing ripe fruit into the world. And this is how it will continue, with those who engage in effective daily spiritual practice continuing to lay the groundwork for the spiritual transformation of all humanity.

We need advaita/non-duality knowledge and the methods of self-inquiry that it provides. This knowledge can bring us inspiration at the beginning of our path, and finally the tools we need when we are ripe and ready to move into the latter stage of our spiritual journey. In-between, most of us have much cultivating to do. Let's recognize that the end stage of our journey to liberation is aided by developing a particular understanding of our nature, what is real versus what is not. But let's not forget that becoming ripe is a prerequisite for developing that understanding. The understanding is experiential, deep within stillness, and not primarily intellectual.

Getting to the stage of ripeness is our responsibility, and it will occur according to our earnest desire (bhakti) and our willingness to keep up our daily practice for as long as it takes. It is important to keep the horse in front of the cart. Then ripeness will surely come, and we will fall off the tree of illusion into the freedom of eternal omnipresent *Oneness*.

Pitfalls of the Mind

The mind is a marvelous machine, capable of performing many great feats of analysis, deduction and discovery. It is also the mind that enables us to create the sense of "*I*" within us. "I am Mary." "I am this body." "I am this mind." "I was born, I am living, and someday I will die."

The end stage of yoga involves using the mind in relationship with our abiding inner silence to question and transcend these deeply rooted assumptions that give rise to the illusory sense of "*I, me, and mine*." Little more is necessary than simply inquiring and releasing in stillness. When we are ready, it will happen automatically.

When combined with the presence of the *witness* resulting from daily deep meditation, inquiries into the nature of our self reveal that we are not our name, our form, or even our sense of "*I*." What we are is the *stillness* behind and within all that is being projected on the screen of our awareness. Our awareness itself is the screen, the only reality. All the rest is a projection that we have become identified with. Ironically, what is seeking within us is the very thing we are seeking.

So, the first pitfall of the mind is *identification*. That is, the identification of our awareness with all the things that are being projected on to it in time and space, including our assumed identity, the "I-ness" and "My-ness" we have assigned to our body, mind and the people and things we hold to be our own. But they are not. It can be a bit scary questioning what we have held as sacred all our life, our sense of self, but as we unwind our identification with objects within and around us, we will find that nothing is destroyed. We will still be here, and all the happier in a vastly more awakened and liberated state.

Indeed, *identification* may be the only pitfall of the mind. Identification of our awareness with this, that or the other thing is at the root of all human foibles and suffering.

The mind has a tendency to ramble on about our life experiences, making up endless *stories*, whether they are in the past, present or future. And the mind will paint them as positive or negative, according to our mood. It is always about one thing – our awareness allowing the mind and associated emotions to wrap us up in something.

Is this the mind's fault? Is there something inherently dysfunctional about the human mind? Or is it something else? After all, the mind is only a machine. Do we blame the automobile when it skids off the road into a tree? Do we blame the hammer when it hits our thumb? Well, maybe some of us do. And perhaps that is a symptom of the underlying problem. If the driver will not take responsibility for the automobile, and the carpenter will not take responsibility for the hammer, then who will? Likewise, if the inhabitant of the mind will not take responsibility for its actions, who will?

Who is the inhabitant of the mind? It is we who are aware, to whatever degree we are aware. The less aware the inhabitant of the mind is, the less likely will the mind be performing as it is designed to, as a servant. Then the mind will be more likely to be operating as a sorcerer's apprentice, feigning leadership as "*I, me, and mine*" and casting a web of conflict and confusion over life. Where there is a vacuum of awareness (the witness not present much) the mind will rush to fill the void with the only thing it can fill it with – lots of thoughts and false perceptions, which are in turn translated to be, "I am these objects of perception…" rather than, "I am the subject, the eternal awareness interpenetrating all these objects…"

So, the first step in helping the mind get back to its rightful purpose is to make sure the inhabitant of the mind will be present and fully awake. This is the *witness*, and we know the prescription by now – daily deep meditation. With the inhabitant of the mind moving in and taking the reins, there will be steady improvement in the operation of the mind. As the clamp of identification is loosened, the functioning of the mind will improve all the way around. There are many practical benefits in this which can be noticed in our daily activities.

But the full integration of inner silence with the mind is not an overnight affair. It takes time. Even with the natural emergence of desire to engage in self-inquiry, there is still a long road to travel to liberation. Along the road there are some particular pitfalls of the mind that may jeopardize our spiritual progress. These are the kinds of pitfalls we'd like to address here, because they can have a bearing on our ability to sustain practices and continued progress on our path:

- Infatuation with or fear of spiritual experiences.
- Over-analyzing and over-philosophizing.
- Overdoing self-inquiry or other yoga practices.
- The illusion of attainment, or of having "arrived."
- Denial of the need to engage in practices.
- The non-duality trap – denying the world as it is.

Such pitfalls of the mind can hamper a spiritual aspirant at any stage along the path. Advanced practitioners are equally susceptible to be drawn off course, perhaps more-so when visited by dramatic experiences of the vastness of pure bliss consciousness, ecstatic bliss, and miraculous powers of one sort or other. These kinds of experiences can rock the mind if inner silence (the *witness*) has not yet been cultivated to a sufficient level of maturity in the nervous system, enabling the practitioner to take advanced spiritual experiences in stride.

So, whether we are just starting out on our path, or are quite far along, cultivating the *witness* will be the best insurance we can have to guard against the pitfalls of the mind.

Infatuation or Fear about Experiences

Spiritual experiences come in many forms and, if we are utilizing effective yoga practices, such experiences will always be associated with purification and opening occurring within us. When experiences come, we will be inclined to think something about them. How we regard them will be a function of our understanding of the processes of yoga and the degree of presence of inner witness we have.

When experience is dramatic, when we are overcome with a large energy flow or a vision of our vastness and *unity* with all things, then we may become identified with the experience. A kind of infatuation can happen then, or even some fear about what we have gotten ourselves into, especially if the internal energy flow becomes excessive, which can lead to a variety of physical and psychological symptoms – also referred to as *kundalini symptoms*.

If we have been approaching our practice from the point of view of our limited self, rather than from the point of view of the witness, we may become infatuated in a way that is similar to romantic infatuation. All infatuations do pass, of course, and in the meantime, we will be wise to favor our practice over the experience. When we are engaged in sitting practices, we can just easily favor the practice we are doing over visions or energy experiences that are coming. If we are in our daily activity, then we can just carry on with our work, whatever it may be.

If experiences overwhelm us to the point where we become fearful that we may be losing control of our life, then it can be helpful to stay engaged in life, particularly in activities that are *grounding*. These are physical activities, and activities that are about engaging with and helping others. At the same time we can temporarily reduce or stop spiritual practices, and, if necessary, the kinds of activities that stimulate spiritual energy flows, such as attending spiritual gatherings, intensive devotional activity, etc. We have mentioned throughout all the AYP writings that this temporary ramping down of spiritual stimulation is called *self-pacing*. Such regulation is a primary consideration in the AYP approach, where an integration of powerful practices is being utilized in a self-directed manner.

Infatuation will pass and fear will subside as inner purification advances and we find a natural integration of the divine within us in everyday living. This is why it is best to carry on with our life, no matter what our spiritual experiences may be. Ultimately, enlightenment is about marrying the spectacular with the ordinary. What remains is *spectacular ordinariness*, which is liberation.

Over-Analyzing and Over-Philosophizing

Whether we are having spiritual experiences or not, constant analysis and philosophizing about our condition (past, present, or future), will not be of much benefit. In fact, this tendency is one of the most common forms of non-relational self-inquiry.

When an experience comes up, whether it be physical, mental, or emotional, we will have a tendency to analyze it. It will be good to understand that taking this to the point of obsession is a common pitfall of the mind.

This doesn't mean we do not analyze or seek confirmation of our path in the scriptures and philosophies that have been written over the centuries. But if we make analysis or philosophy the object of our path, we will be veering off on a tangent that can undermine our commitment to yoga practices and developing our ability in relational self-inquiry. When analysis and philosophy creep up to the point where they become ends in themselves, then we have entered into the realm of building castles in the air, which is non-relational and not effective spiritual practice.

In that case, we can just observe and let go of the excessive analysis in favor of cultivating the witness in our sitting practices, and going out and living our life fully.

Overdoing Self-Inquiry or other Yoga Practices

A common pitfall of the mind is found in the idea that if a little of a particular practice is bringing us some results, then a lot more of it will bring even more results.

For example, if we have asked ourselves, "Who am I?" and a flash of inspiration comes, we might conclude that we should be asking ourselves "Who am I?" twenty-four hours per day, seven days per week.

Likewise, if we have been engaging in daily deep meditation twice each day for twenty minutes (a balanced practice), and find a noticeable presence of the inner witness coming up, then we might conclude that meditating much longer and more often will be better.

In either case (non-stop self-inquiry or non-stop deep meditation), we will be stepping into a mental pitfall that can actually slow our spiritual progress.

Overdoing practices will only produce excessive purification and strain that will limit our ability to practice effectively until balance has returned.

While some teachers preach the possibility of instant enlightenment, that all we are is here and now, it does in fact take some time to open up the nervous system to our greater possibilities within. It is a process which can be accelerated in particular ways, but not on a flight of fancy that more is always going to be better. The path to enlightenment involves a process of *purification and opening* that takes time, depending on our long term consistency in practices and the internal matrix of obstructions being dissolved in our nervous system. No matter what methods we are following, there are few if any shortcuts that can bypass the need for *self-pacing* in practices.

Rome was not built in a day; and neither is the process of human spiritual transformation completed in a day. If we are steadfast in applying tried and true methods over time, the result will be there. The journey to enlightenment is a marathon, not a sprint.

The Illusion of Attainment or of Having Arrived

Enlightenment, the direct realization of who we are, is unassuming and does not proclaim itself, except by compassionate assistance offered for the benefit of others. Conversely, where there is the assumption of attainment or of having arrived, actions can be distorted accordingly, leading to a rigid teaching, proselytizing, sectarianism, and a shift in focus from spiritual practices to the one who has supposedly arrived. It is a common pitfall of the mind that may be found lurking in the teacher, the student, or both.

When consciousness is identified with the mind, there will be a great need to proclaim victory over the forces of ignorance. This breeds more ignorance, of course. There can be no enlightenment proclaimed on the level of the mind. The functioning of the mind can only be seen as a symptom of the illumination which comes from within, or the lack of it. We may conclude that an inner flow is occurring, or not, but we can never proclaim with accuracy that we have arrived, for that is beyond the province of the mind.

By definition, both the cause and the destination of true realization are beyond the mind, in the abiding inner witness, which never assumes or proclaims anything. It just is.

When there is some proclaiming going on, it is wise to ask, "Who is proclaiming?" and then let it go in stillness.

Denying Practices

There are rare cases of individuals who reach what seems to be an enlightened state in this life with little or no effort in spiritual practices. Or perhaps they have forgotten? It is natural for such individuals to promote the idea of enlightenment requiring no practices from their point of view. They routinely will say, "There is nothing to do. You are there already."

It is like the New Yorker who mysteriously wakes up in California one day, not knowing how he got there, and then calling all his friends in New York to tell them they can do the same. If only…

This kind of teaching is flawed, to say the least. While the destination may be true, the means will be lacking for nearly everyone. So, when a teacher tells us that we need do nothing to reach enlightenment, and we do not find ourselves there in that instant, then it will be wise to review additional means that are available. In this case the conclusion of the enlightened one is a mental pitfall (yes, they do have them), and to follow such a teaching to the exclusion of everything else is a mental pitfall in the student.

A common symptom of the illusion of having arrived can be a loss of recognition of the value of spiritual practices. It is one of the greatest risks for advanced practitioners – falling into the belief that our journey to realization is done. The next thought the mind will produce is, "I don't have to practice any more." And wherever we happen to be on the path at that point, that is more or less where we will stay until we wake up enough to realize that our spiritual progress never ends, and therefore the need for spiritual practice will never end either. Practices may change according to our ongoing purification and opening, but the need for them will never end.

This is not to imply that all practices that are available in a system like AYP ought to be undertaken in a rigid way. Our application of practices will always be tempered by *self-pacing* to accommodate our personal inclinations and capacity for purification and opening, which can change over time. This measured approach to practice, or even no practice in times of rapid purification and opening, is obviously not the same as a blanket instruction to shun all spiritual practices in favor of direct realization, which will not be in tune with the individual needs of many on the path.

The reason there is no end on the path is because there is no such thing as individual enlightenment in the ultimate sense. As we are approaching individual enlightenment, we begin to know ourselves to be all that is around us. Then the condition of consciousness of all who are around us is seen to be our condition. So we will not be fully enlightened until everyone is enlightened. This is why so-called enlightened people continue to work for the benefit of all. Their liberation will not be fulfilled until everyone's is. And neither shall ours. There is much joy and fulfillment to be found along the way, as long as we continue with our practices, yielding ever-increasing expansion to the infinite! Long before we reach that infinite stage, we will be free.

The Non-Duality Trap – Denying the World

Sages may tell us that the world is not real, but only a projection occurring via our senses and the perception of objects through the identification of our awareness. On the other hand, it has been said that perception is 100% of reality, and this is also true.

Our reality is what we perceive it to be. But the sage will say that it is all illusion, and that if we deconstruct the machinery of the identification of our awareness with our perceptions, we will find that there is nothing here at all.

Well, true. We learned it in high school quantum physics. All of existence is empty space with infinitesimal bits of energy moving in it. Does our limited identified sense of self have any meaning in this vast realm of emptiness? It can be argued that it is all meaningless. But is this a useful view of our world? Can we continue to function with such a view when taken on the level of the intellect alone? Not likely. Happily, there is much more, but we can't get there with the intellect alone.

While the logic of non-duality is impeccable, the assumption that it can be realized instantly by everyone is incorrect. Teachers who disregard the perceptions of others (100% of their reality) and refuse to meet them where they are will fail to help them. In fact, damage can be done by encouraging students to reach far beyond where they are perceptually without offering intermediate steps.

We know that if we try to run before we have learned to walk, we will land flat on our face, and may find ourselves in serious trouble with our motivation and ability to function in the world. For most practitioners of self-inquiry, laboring to deny the existence of the world is destructive. While we can certainly find inspiration in the concept of *Oneness*, to attempt to live that in the mind is a huge pitfall. This is because Oneness (non-duality) is not of the mind. As soon as we try and live it there, we will find much of our life to be meaningless and nihilistic, experiencing a false rejection of everyday living, and this is very unhealthy. This is non-relational self-inquiry at its worst.

The paradox in this is that the experience of *Oneness* is highly meaningful in all aspects of life, and is the source of all love and sharing in *unity*. The non-dual condition is an experience of *unity*, of radiant love and joining, not an experience of separation – not a denial of the world at all. It is liberation in this life.

If we are doing self-inquiry with the presence of the *witness*, we will not fall into the trap of denying life as it is. Instead we will find ourselves coming more and more into the condition of becoming life as it is, which can also be described as being in the world but not of the world. This is real *Oneness*, real non-duality, real *advaita-vedanta*, the fruit of yoga, and of *jnana yoga* in particular. It is not the divisive non-relational kind of self-inquiry that can lead to years of struggle and misery. There is a much better way of affirming the sacred proclamation of the sages that "All are *One*."

Or, as we say in AYP, "The *One* is the many and the many are the *One*."

Chapter 3 – Undoing The Doer

The primary cause of suffering in this life is not pain, whether it be physical, mental or emotional. There will be pain for sure. It is inevitable. But we will only suffer if we are living in a mode where we are *identified* with that experience. While we cannot immediately will ourselves to cease being identified with our pain, we can gradually reduce our identification through spiritual practices, until one day we are no longer suffering at all, even when going through the many ups and downs of life.

On a seemingly more abstract level, we can say that this process of reducing identification with the objects of perception is *undoing the doer*.

Who is the doer? The doer is simply whoever or whatever we perceive ourselves to be. The doer is not a fixed entity. In fact, as we become advanced in our spiritual practices and experiences, we will find that the doer is no entity at all, nowhere to be found as "*I, me, or mine*," but something vast and universal that is flowing through us and all around us in this realm of time and space. This is not theory, at least not in the discussions we prefer to have in relation to the AYP system of practices. Rather, it is *experiential*.

What we find as we continue to practice daily is that our sense of doership gradually shifts from an *egocentric awareness* identified with the body-mind to a separate unshakable sense of *silent witness* residing within us, and finally to a sense of *eternal Oneness* flowing spontaneously through all of life, including through all that we are and do as human beings. This is the journey of human spiritual transformation, and the path to freedom in this life.

Undoing the doer is not a war on the ego. It is a transformation of ego via a blissful expansion of our sense of self from a very limited level of identification with the objects of perception, including our body-mind and all experiences, to an infinite view that encompasses everything, without being trapped in the clutches of identified awareness.

Role and Evolution of the Witness

The first step on this journey once our fire of desire for liberation has been kindled is to cultivate abiding inner silence, which we will notice as the quality of witnessing in all that we experience and do. With a twice-daily routine of deep meditation, the rise of the witness is inevitable.

With the witness, we will notice that all objects of perception will begin to appear outside our sense of self, including our thoughts and feelings. This provides a unique opportunity to conduct our life from a deeper place within us, a place that does not identify itself with the ups and downs of mundane existence. In this condition, our sense of self has shifted from object-based, to stillness-based. Our sense of being the doer has shifted also, from a physical being to an abiding inner silent witness.

This sense of witnessing enables us to look further into the nature of life and our role in it. In time, we begin to see that we have been viewing the witness itself as an object of perception. Then we will see our sense of self moving beyond the witness to something that is not definable as an object at all. Then we use words like *dispassion* and *unity* to describe the doing. But what we really mean is that it is out of our personal hands, as we are engaging fully and effectively in daily life in a state of *active surrender* to the flow within and around us.

Here is a progression that shows how the witness plays its role in our spiritual unfoldment as we engage in daily deep meditation and related practices. In time, the witness is dissolved as an object in our infinite awareness and our sense of self goes beyond:

- Pre-Witnessing – Information and intellectual assessments about truth provide inspiration, and a tendency to build mental castles in the air, ideas reacting with ideas, which is not spiritually progressive. So we do what is necessary to cultivate the witness.

- Witnessing – Perceiving the world, our thoughts and feelings as objects separate from our sense of self in stillness. It is the beginning of progressive spiritual inquiry and growth, consciously chosen or not.

- Discrimination – The reversal of identification with the objects of perception occurs by logical choices based on direct perception rooted in stillness. This is a more advanced application of the witness which is able to discern the real from the unreal, and begins to take us beyond the witness as an object of perception.

- Dispassion – Rise of the condition of no judgment and no attachment (including to the witness state). The process of spiritual unfoldment becomes automatic to the point of all objects being constantly dissolved in an ocean of stillness, like waves on the surface of the sea are naturally reabsorbed. It is the unwinding of identification.

- Unity – The merging of subject and object: "I am *That*. You are *That*. All this is *That*." Ongoing outpouring divine love and service to others as universal *Self*. It is *liberation*.

While progress on the road to enlightenment may be erratic, difficult, or non-existent when engaged in self-inquiry as a stand-alone approach, it is quite a different story when self-inquiry is used in concert with a path based on an integration of tried and true yoga methods.

The cultivation of inner silence (the witness) in deep meditation assures that our perception will be expanding from within over time, and this provides for an increasingly fertile field for the process of self-inquiry to occur. So too, does our experience in daily samyama practice cultivate our ability to release in stillness and live more from the level of our abiding inner silence.

As purification and opening proceed within us, our self-inquiry methods will change and refine over time, as we migrate from pre-witnessing to witnessing, discrimination, dispassion and *unity*.

The steady emergence of inner silence and our ability to release our intentions and perceptions within it are the dynamics behind the progression of self-inquiry from non-relational to relational, until the experiencer and the experience have merged to become *One*, self-sufficient, active in the world, and free of the bondage of identification and suffering.

Pre-Witnessing

How meaningful is self-inquiry of the absolute (non-duality) kind when we are still in the pre-witnessing stage of mind? This is when all things are still considered primarily on the level of thinking and logic. In this state, what does it mean to us when we hear, "All this you see here in the world is illusion, and you are the reality behind it."

We might have some inspiration, a desire may be kindled to know more, to be more. Hopefully. But the more we think about it, the more layers we will create around that essential desire to know the truth. How many times will we have to repeat the question "Who am I?" before we will have a glimmer of who and what we really are? And how many books will we have to read? This is why we call pre-witnessing the stage of inspiration and building castles in the air. Not much more than this can happen until we move to the next stage. With suitable inspiration, we will be compelled to take action beyond pounding the idea against the infinite with our tiny brain! The mind can only run in circles for so long before we realize that we must add something else to the mix. Once we are inspired to uncover the truth, it is important to take action, intelligent action.

Non-duality purists will say, "Take no action. Do nothing. Just be!"

Well, we can attempt to do that for a very long time in pre-witnessing mode. No doubt we can develop some witness quality by working on just being. But there is a much faster way.

If we commit to take action using all the tools that are available to us, we can travel quickly along the road of realizing what we already are – our inner-most immovable *Self.* With deep meditation and a full battery of supporting practices we will move surely into the witnessing stage.

Witnessing

The witnessing stage is a whole new ball game. It should be pointed out that there is a continuum of development as witnessing emerges. It begins as a passive inner condition perceived as a separation from the events going on around us, often first noticed during the occurrence of dynamic events. Everyone has had the experience of "time standing still" when a dynamic event occurred, like a car crash, explosion or other sudden change in our physical environment. When the witness begins to emerge, ordinary events are gradually experienced more in this way also. As witnessing continues to advance, our body, thoughts and feelings become objects of perception that are separate from our sense of self, our witness. This is an important development.

Before the witness has developed to the point where our thoughts and feelings become objects of perception, self-inquiry will be mostly non-relational, meaning not fully connected with who we are – pure consciousness. The dawn of the witness sets the stage for real self-inquiry, and an ongoing change in our life experience, for this is when the process can move beyond ideas to the direct experience. And the direct experience is *beyond* all experience. In the initial witness condition, we are experiencing, but we are not the experience. We are beyond it, seeing from the point of view of separate pure awareness.

There are a few more steps beyond the emergence of the witness that we must go through. It is not enough to be strongly established in inner silence, seeing the changing world as separate from ourselves. We must do something with it to move it forward. Evolution compels us to do so. With a little nudging, it happens naturally enough. This is where self-inquiry can have its greatest impact on our overall path to enlightenment, because we are able to make conscious choices based in our stillness. We see our thoughts, feelings and perceptions of the world for what they are, without being entirely identified with them. We are then able to engage in a way that is liberating rather than binding, both for ourselves and for others.

Other yoga practices are an aid to this process, such as samyama, spinal breathing pranayama, and additional practices that cultivate ecstatic conductivity (kundalini awakening) in the body. As we become more established in both inner silence and ecstatic conductivity, we experience refinements in perception and the movement of dynamic stillness into our thought processes. These developments support steadily increasing effectiveness in relational self-inquiry.

Discrimination

When we think of discrimination, the normal interpretation is that we are choosing between this or that thing – choosing between this or that idea. Non-relational self-inquiry is like that, choosing between things, ideas, and ways we imagine we would like for life to be. This kind of discrimination is circular, goes nowhere fast, and may go nowhere for a long time. Even choosing not to think is a gigantic task when undertaken non-relationally, without the witness present to support our endeavor.

With the rising presence of the witness, the entire dynamic of self-inquiry changes. Then we are choosing between that which is object (things, ideas, and emotions) and that which is subject (witness, or *Self*). And that kind of choosing is not a doing at all. It is a letting go. It is a surrender, even while we are being active in the world.

We all know what we want. We want to know the truth. We want to be happy. We want to be free. Since childhood we have been told that the truth will set us free from the burdens of this life. So we want *That*.

As the witness becomes more and more abiding and we are quietly observing every thought and feeling from that perspective, we come to know ourselves as *That*, unshaken and independent of all of our experiences, including our own thoughts. Then we are finally in the position to make choices that will unwind the habitual identification with experiences and the dream we have been living in up until now.

It is a new perspective from which we can clearly see what is real and what is not. At the same time, it is both as profound and as simple as directly perceiving what is eternal and what is not. And we can discriminate accordingly, making logical choices that are grounded in stillness, unwinding the lingering habit of the mind to identify itself with the objects of experience, both outside and inside us.

In the language of *advaita* (non-duality), it is called "neti neti," which means *not this, not this*. When the witness is sufficiently present for relational self-inquiry to occur in the form of discrimination, then neti neti becomes a reality. We directly perceive what is true and what is not, and we can easily choose, including choosing what is our greater *Self* over what is not (*I, me, and mine*).

Before our discrimination becomes relational (in stillness), neti neti will be an exercise of the intellect, and will be as ineffective and exhausting as any other form of non-relational self-inquiry. We will know the witness is dawning in earnest when discrimination becomes easier. It is a telltale sign.

A certain excitement comes with the realization that we have arrived at the point of being able to choose with certainty that which is real over that which is not. There can even be an enthusiasm to the exclusion of all else, and we have to guard against throwing out the practices that have brought us to this point. There can be a tendency to plant our flag on the notion that we are *That*, and fixate on the idea that all we have to do from then on is hang onto *That*.

If this happens, it can be slipping into non-relational self-inquiry again. It is one of those pitfalls of the mind we discussed earlier. It can happen to advanced practitioners. Much better we should continue with the practices that brought us to this point and strengthen the presence of the witness beyond all tendencies we might have to imagine that we have attained anything. Even the most advanced practitioners must guard against falling into non-relational self-inquiry.

Certainly we can take giant leaps toward realization when our ability has risen to clearly discriminate between objects (external and internal) and the subject (the witness – our *Self*). It is prime time for self-inquiry. But it will not be the only thing going on, assuming we have been wise and continue with our daily routine of yoga practices. All methods combined will assure our rapid forward progress.

Self-inquiry is useful, but it cannot be trusted to operate alone. Certainly not at the discrimination stage, or at any prior stage.

There will come a time when discrimination begins to give way to something else. It is the letting go of the need to make choices anymore. The subject (witness) becomes so well-established that choices no longer need to be made. We just are, and we can allow everything in our field of awareness to just be, even as we are interacting normally in everyday living. We call this the dispassion stage. It is the stage of being completely unruffled by anything that happens inside or outside us.

Dispassion

The condition of dispassion is one of the primary goals of self-inquiry and of all of yoga. Those who are very enthusiastic and dedicated to self-inquiry are very passionate about developing dispassion. This is non-relational self-inquiry, of course. We all have to begin somewhere. We can't begin at the end, though we may certainly be passionate about the ideal we have chosen, and that serves a purpose. It is our bhakti (devotion to our chosen ideal).

Dispassion is not a doing at all, and is beyond all inquiry. It isn't even a letting go, for it is beyond choice. Dispassion is a state of being. It is the subject (the witness, our sense of *Self*) developed through an integration of practices to the point where all the objects of experience are taken in stride, without identification. This applies to events, relationships, and all that is going on in the body, heart and mind, including the witness itself as an object of perception.

Is dispassion a state of indifference, a state of uncaring? Does it mean we do not act or react in the world? It does not mean that. It is just the opposite – the rise of dispassion corresponds with the rise of compassion. Much of spiritual development is paradoxical like that, with less becoming much more.

The gradual emergence of dispassion means we are becoming more free to act for the good of all. Inner silence will *move* to do this through us more and more, the further we travel along the path. It is the paradox of enlightenment. The more we have gone beyond, the more engaged we will become for the benefit of others. This is the nature of divine consciousness.

We really have to give credit where credit is due. Deep meditation (if we are doing it) is the primary cultivator of dispassion, because dispassion is an advanced stage of the witness – in fact, the witness going beyond itself, beyond *Self*. As long as there is a sense of *Self*, there is duality. *Unity* is beyond sense of *Self*, even as we are acting in the world as though we are seeing the world as an extension of our own *Self*. It is a paradox.

A stand-alone path of self-inquiry can lead to dispassion also, but it is rare. To succeed, a stand alone approach to self-inquiry must ascend to the level of meditation, the transcendence of all objects of attention. If self-inquiry is done like this over time, then the witness will dawn and, in more time, there will be dispassion. It is a difficult path, because it lacks a structured and efficient routine of practice. The concept of *practice* itself may be lacking. Self-inquiry of the stand-alone variety will be about constantly remembering to release all objects of perception, including all thoughts, feelings and perceptions of external objects. When such self-inquiry becomes a deeply ingrained habit, then that will be a kind of ongoing meditation. How an approach like this will fit into daily life is another question, since it requires ongoing self-inquiry to be incorporated into every nook and cranny of our daily life. This may not be practical for someone with a family and career. There can be direct conflicts, particularly before the witness has dawned.

On the other hand, if deep meditation and other sitting practices are undertaken in a structured twice-daily routine, and life is lived normally, the witness will be coming up naturally as a support to family and career, and also as a support to undertake self-inquiry in a way that does not disrupt the normal flow of life. Deep meditation provides the witness, and self-inquiry (supported by samyama and the ability to inquire relationally in stillness) provides the perspective in a way that is not replacing everyday life and activities, but enhancing them.

Dispassion is at home in the marketplace, as well as in the remote retreat. It is all the same. The combination of daily deep meditation and gradually emerging self-inquiry provides flexibility for living, and is a much faster path as well.

Unity

No one knows what the true nature of existence is outside the realm of time and space. Yet, oddly enough, we can experience it directly. The reason we say "We cannot know" is because the reality we are able to experience through deep meditation and self-inquiry is outside the field of knowing. It is *That*, and thousands of volumes have been written attempting to describe *That*.

In the end, the best we can do is say, "I am *That*." Then we can carry on with the many descriptions of *That* – pure bliss consciousness, void, Tao, God, Allah… It doesn't really matter what we call it. *That* is as good a word as any, and we are *That*. All that exists is *That*.

If it sounds a little impersonal, it is not intended to be. For *That* is the source of all love, compassion, goodness, creativity and happiness in the world. *That* illuminates us with these divine qualities, and is the source of all good deeds.

There is a misunderstanding that has been perpetuated by some teachers – the premise that becoming *That* is the only thing of importance and nothing here on earth matters at all. In fact, according to this premise, nothing here on earth exists. In a purely philosophical sense this may be true. Yet, when taken on the level of intellect, it is one of the biggest traps for getting stuck in non-relational self-inquiry.

There is the idea that it matters not one bit what becomes of this earth or the multitude of life that is on it. There is a distinction between one who is truly enlightened and one who has created a division between themselves and the rest of the world through non-relational self-inquiry, enforced by a rigid intellectual view. With clear relational self-inquiry based in stillness, we can reject this out of hand. Neti neti!

The enlightened one will be he or she who remains engaged for the benefit of all, as *That*. Advancement on the path to enlightenment brings with it the perception that we can only be free when all are free, for we are *One* with all who are suffering.

The image of the lone sage on the mountaintop, indifferent to the travails of the world, is fiction. If a sage is not engaged in some way for the benefit of others, their condition will be in question. True enlightenment is the spontaneous outpouring of divine love, which is working constantly to uplift everyone. The true sage becomes a willing and wide open channel for *That*, which does nothing even while doing everything.

So, while yoga and self-inquiry are often viewed as a going beyond, never to return, it is not so. We can never leave what is here and now, for it is what we are in our own *Self*. The journey of yoga, and of self-inquiry, is a journey beyond all that is, including, paradoxically, any sense of *Self*, ending in a return and full engagement for the betterment of humankind – a journey from *here to here*. This is the highest knowledge, and its highest manifestation in this world. By the time we have gone beyond *Self*, we can only call it *That*:

"I am *That*. You are *That*. All this is *That*."

It is an unending outpouring of divine love, whose fundamental nature and ultimate fruition is life everywhere flowing in the *Oneness* of *unity*. It has always been *That* and will always be *That*. The witness and self-inquiry lead to direct realization of *That* in this life.

What about I, Me, and Mine?

If we look at all of this from the point of view of the *ego*, the role and evolution of the *witness* we have just described is not only the undoing of suffering and the doer, but also the undoing of the limited idea of "*I, me, and mine*." By "limited idea," we mean that our sense of "*I*" is a mental construct embedded deep within the mind, and not a real thing at all. It is a state of self-imposed limitation and bondage we live in, and the dissolution of it is at the core of end stage liberation.

This isn't to say that the ego is not our friend. It certainly is when it comes to any sort of spiritual practice, and for getting along in the world too. We can only operate from the sense of self that we have, and from that level we make choices to practice meditation, pranayama, self-inquiry and other methods that lead us to freedom. It is the ego that is sawing off the limb it is sitting on, so it can be dissolved in the eternity of pure bliss consciousness. Even then, the ego enables us to function in the world with essential things like making a living, doing for others, etc.

In the AYP approach, we do not see the ego, nor the mind, as adversaries or enemies. Rather, we see them as vehicles to a fuller life, our allies on the journey. Without them, we could not travel forward one inch from where we are. By recognizing the ego as the doer when we are starting out, we are able to sit and meditate, cultivate the witness, and do all the rest that leads us to freedom.

It is likewise with the *witness*. Some teachers, in addition to denigrating the ego and the mind, pooh pooh the witness, saying that it is an incomplete stage of development, because it may be viewed as the subject separate from the objects of perception. The criticism is that the witness is perceived as an object, and an object cannot be the subject, so the witness is not end stage enlightenment. True, but can we skip over any stage of development? We must decide as ego to practice, and then next discover as witness how to loosen the bonds of identification of awareness with the objects of perception, including the witness. Then we go beyond the witness as we enter the non-dual condition. And so it goes, step-by-step.

Subject, Object, and the Mechanics of Perception

Let's take a look at the structure of things – the *witness* and its relationship to our *sense of self*, the mechanics of perception, and the objects of perception. It is this relationship that we seek to enliven in a way that enables us to move beyond the limitations of time and space, and the suffering that is inherent in the human condition, even while remaining fully human and engaged in life for the betterment and happiness of all.

Since the beginning of the AYP writings, from the time when we first provided instructions for deep meditation, we have used various phrases to describe what we are cultivating with our practice – abiding inner silence, stillness, pure bliss consciousness, sat-chit-ananda, the witness, etc. All of these add up to the same thing – an increasing sense of calmness, steadiness and peace coming up behind our sensory perceptions, thoughts, feelings and activities in the world. At some point we notice that, while everything within and around us is moving, something fundamental within us is not moving. We have called it "*the witness*." So steady is this silent awareness, that we also have recognized it as being at the root of our sense of self. Even so, we have still been in duality with the witness, meaning we are "in here" as the immovable witness, and at the same time "out there" involved in everything that is in motion, including our thoughts, feelings, sensory perceptions and action in the world, all of which are external to the witness.

While we know ourselves to be separate, we have also known ourselves to be in the world of our body-mind and everything else. So our sense of self, our "*I-sense*," is divided into "*me*" unmoving in here, and "*me*" still engaged in everything out there. It is a condition of duality. This sense of duality actually becomes amplified when we first notice our witness quality, because we sense ourselves alone and separate from the events occurring within and around us. This amplified sense of duality in early witness stage is normal and only temporary, as we shall see.

The duality we experience in everyday life is found in the dynamic of the observer (subject), the process of observation (perception), and object of observation. It is "*me*" and "*the other*" – two, or dual. Before the witness (pre-witnessing stage of mind discussed earlier), the observer was considered to be the body-mind, as in, "I am the body-mind observing these objects." In this situation, the subject ("*I*") is identified as an object. It is the object (body-mind) masquerading as subject and viewing other objects – an object-to-object duality. This is the stickiness of awareness, identifying itself with an object, the body-mind, creating a false sense of self, what we call *ego*. Awareness is so sticky that we may even consider our possessions to be extensions of our self – my house, my car, my money, my family, my nation, etc. The consequences of this kind of self-identification are well known. Just read today's news headlines that chronicle the foibles of *"I, me, and mine"* operating all around the world for its own perceived interests. Surely we can do better.

With the witness coming up, all of this object identification begins to recede, enough so that while we may still feel we are the body-mind, we also know that we are beyond it in abiding inner silence. It is still duality, but a more liberated kind of duality, and this begins to be noticed in our perceptions and actions. It is our deeper sense of *Self* (witness) seeing objects instead of a limited ego self seeing objects. It is a big step forward that can enhance the quality of our life dramatically. As we experience the abiding witness, it is the experience of duality in transition to *unity*.

Taking it to the point where our sense of self is able to release entirely from identification with the body-mind and other objects of perception is the next step. It is a step that can take some time of gradual uncoupling of the self-identification (stickiness) of awareness. The more gradual the uncoupling, the more stable and lasting the result will be. Some have claimed the uncoupling to happen suddenly, with or without measures taken beforehand to stimulate it.

Sudden transformations of self-identification are possible. They are often accompanied by physical and psychological trials, and repeated setbacks. Rome was not built in a day, but one way or another it will be built! In the AYP approach, with the full range of practices we have available to us, we have been cultivating the *witness* directly in deep meditation, and begun moving stillness with samyama and basic forms of self-inquiry. With all of this, our sense of self has been slowly receding from the objects of perception, including the body-mind.

During this gradual receding of self-identification with objects, the relationship of observer, process of observation, and objects of observation remains intact. It does not change. What changes is our sense of self, our *I-sense*. It moves out gradually from the objects of perception into our emerging unbounded awareness. As it does, the initial duality between the witness and the objects of perception becomes gradually less dual and more non-dual. This means that the two, witness and objects, gradually become *One*. With the loosening of identification of our awareness with the objects of perception, our sense of self expands to become increasingly universal, not tied to any particular object, but found to be underlying all objects; no longer self-identified with objects, but underlying them in a way that we no longer see ourselves as being in the world, but instead, the world being in us. At that time we are justified in replacing the small "s" in self with a big "*S*." We have gone from being a small identified self, to being the big universal *Self*. This is not philosophical. It is experiential. It is not a concept we can manifest as reality via the mind. It is a neurobiological condition that we find ourselves living in 24 hours per day, as a result of effective practices engaged in over time.

As this shift occurs, it can be said that we are moving *beyond the witness*, because we are no longer observing objects as being outside ourselves, including the witness. Even as everything is still moving, we do not see it moving, and this is the condition of no objects – subject only. What we see is stillness moving, only *One*, a paradox for sure, a different experience than the two of observer and observed. The mechanics of perception are still operating as before within this rising unified non-dual experience. What has changed is our sense of self in relation to all of that. What we see, no matter what we are looking at, is only *Self*, or *That*. The duality of observer, process of observation, and object of observation is still functioning, but it has become transparent to us, much the way the detailed functioning of many aspects of nature are already transparent to us, including the multitude of activities occurring automatically within our physical body. We see the whole body and not the millions of activities that are occurring within it. Like that, as we become consciously the whole of infinite awareness, we may barely notice the many events that are occurring within our *Self*, including the body-mind. We engage and we are involved, but our sense of self is beyond the details, which are spontaneously expressing radiating divine love coming from our omnipresent center, our *Self*. We are *That*.

But we are not going to be completely transformed to this condition of freedom and divine radiance in a single day, or even in a single year. It is a process, a journey, first to the *witness* stage, and then moving steadily beyond the witness stage into *Oneness*. Along the way the temporal world as we have known it gradually dissolves in the pure light of *Being*, even while we have gone nowhere, and not even changed our daily routine of activities. It has always been like that. We just have not realized it until we went through the process of purification, opening and awakening. It is a journey from *here to here*.

The Techniques of Jnana Yoga

Assuming we are up for it, having a burning desire to be liberated from the suffering of self-identified awareness, let's see what can be done to move this natural progression along. Indeed, many have been clamoring for more as the witness has been rising in everyone, particularly those who have been engaged in daily practices over the years.

The methods we are looking at here are called *jnana yoga*, which means the yoga of experiential knowledge. It is the same as *advaita-vedanta*, which is the knowledge of the non-dual nature of life. Vedanta means *"the end of the knowledge,"* which is end stage human spiritual transformation.

The logical approach has been to first attack the problem with the mind, which in many cases turns out to be like appointing the bandit to be the policeman. Not that there is anything wrong with the mind. But if we are still self-identified with the mind, thinking that "I am doing this," even with some presence of the witness, forward progress will be difficult. The mind has its limitations. Without a deeper connection occurring in stillness, the mind will be like a tail trying to wag a big dog. It won't happen. What we need is abiding inner silence. Then it becomes easy to utilize means that enable us to slip through the snares of the intellect and the castles in the air it is inclined to build when left to its own devices.

In other words, liberation is not primarily an intellectual challenge. Pure intellectuals are certainly the worst-equipped for self-inquiry, the primary tool of *jnana yoga* and *advaita-vedanta*. Rather, it is a journey of the *witness* in relation to everything else, necessarily with the application of specific mental techniques as the aspirant is becoming *ripe*. It is much the way deep meditation and spinal breathing pranayama involve the use of specific mental techniques that enable us to transcend the mind and its objects, cultivating the core qualities of enlightenment – abiding stillness and ecstasy.

Now we want to merge these core qualities and move onward through the stages of discrimination, dispassion and *unity*. In this way, we can go beyond the witness stage. For this, we have taken an important step if we have added structured daily samyama practice into our daily routine. This cultivates in us the habit of releasing intentions and inquiries in stillness, making everything we do more fluid in expressing the divine flow in all aspects of our life. Once we have developed the habit of samyama (moving in stillness), we find ourselves in an excellent position to travel the road of relational self-inquiry. That is, inquiry in stillness.

Previously, we have discussed the evolving stages of our awareness as witness, and the applications of the mind in relation to our emerging abiding inner silence. We can expand on these in terms of *jnana yoga*, and categorize them in this way:

- **Jnana-Natural** – Through sitting practices, the rise of the witness and dissolving of self-identification with objects via unstructured (natural) self-inquiry in daily activity.

- **Jnana-Releasing** – Systematic methods utilizing inquiry and discrimination for the release of non-evolutionary thoughts and feelings: "I choose to question the truth of my thoughts, and release that which is untrue."

- **Jnana-Affirming** – Affirmation of our nature as *One* and the same as eternal *Self/God* through our chosen ideal: "I am *That*."

- **Jnana-Negating** – Discrimination using negation of identification with all objects of perception, including all thoughts and feelings for *Self*-realization: "Not this, not this" (neti neti).

- **Jnana-Transcending** – Inquiring directly into what our "I-sense" is, releasing it into its source (witness) for *Self*-realization: "Who am I?"

There may be significant overlap between these in any given system of practice, or in the preferences of the practitioner. In considering these categories of self-inquiry, the thing to take note of is where we are on our path right now, and how that resonates with the variety of inquiry methods available. The goal is not to jump immediately to the method furthest down the list, but to find one that resonates with our current condition. By "resonates," we mean it improves our sense of wellbeing (however we perceive that), without making a mess of it. For many who are coming to self-inquiry with serious intentions for the first time, the method will be *jnana-natural* leading into *jnana-releasing*, which are concerned with practical self-inquiry addressing our immediate issues in everyday living. That is where it begins for most of us.

Jnana-Natural

With a daily routine of effective yoga practices, we will find abiding inner silence coming up, more experience of witnessing, and an increasing fluidity of our thoughts, feelings and actions flowing out from stillness on the wings of rising ecstatic conductivity and radiance. What to think about all this as it is happening? We will obviously be thinking something about it as we go about our daily life. In time, we come to realize that our sense of self is shifting naturally from the objects of perception to this inner silence that has arisen underneath all of our life experiences, including our inner processes of perception, thinking and feeling. It is quite easy to go with that shift in our *I-sense*, and this is what we can call the advent of natural *advaita* – natural non-duality. It is also natural *jnana yoga*, which is the same thing.

Recall that all the limbs of yoga are connected, so it is not out of the ordinary for progress in one area of yoga to stimulate progress in other areas of yoga. The more areas of yoga we are engaged in, the more synergies will be arising, and the more rapid our progress. The wisdom inherent within us (our inner guru) knows this, so as we find natural non-duality arising, we will be inclined to inquire. It can be an intuitive kind of inquiring occurring as we go about our daily business – something as simple as, "Who is it having this experience?" and release. It can take many forms, limited only by our imagination.

<u>The underlying feature in all true self-inquiry is that it is released in stillness.</u>

This ability is what we have been developing in our structured samyama practice all along. With daily deep meditation and samyama, relational self-inquiry (in stillness) is inevitable. The rise of the witness and our ability to release our intentions in it is the foundation of effective self-inquiry.

Along the way, we may be inspired to add more structured forms of self-inquiry. How we go about it will depend on our personal inclinations. Even if we do not have strong bhakti (spiritual desire) for a far-reaching ideal of non-duality, styles of self-inquiry that deal with the issues we encounter in daily life are very effective and will lead us forward. It is an easy place to start, and brings practical benefits in the here and now, in our relationships, in our work, and in the increasingly illuminated way that we see the world in general. With the witness, we begin to see our thoughts and feelings as objects, and in doing so we find ourselves with the option to release or transform inner patterns to support our best interests. In time, this will have far-reaching implications. All of this occurs naturally through us as a result of daily yoga practices.

Jnana-Releasing

With abiding inner silence (the witness) coming up, our thoughts and feelings increasingly are perceived as the objects of perception that they are. Before that, we may have identified with these perceptions as our self, taking our thoughts and feelings more seriously than was for our own good.

The first step on the road to traveling beyond duality (subject and object) in witness stage is a deepening of our understanding of thoughts/feelings (including our sense of "*I, me, and mine*") being not the same as our *Self*. With daily deep meditation, this will begin as a natural realization. If we choose to take a more active role, we can engage in more structured practical inquiry into our everyday thoughts and feelings, releasing and/or transforming them to improve the quality of our life. At the same time, this kind of everyday inquiry will, over time, move us gradually toward the non-dual condition of *unity*.

The popular styles of releasing techniques that are out there, systematically questioning our thoughts and feelings in daily life, offer practical self-inquiry, and have been shown to be effective over the years. Systems of this kind are a good starting point for practitioners looking to undertake a basic form of structured self-inquiry. That is assuming abiding inner silence (the witness) is being cultivated.

The *jnana-releasing* style of self-inquiry involves inquiring into and making conscious choices about our thoughts and feelings, regarding them as objects. An inquiry can be about the truth of a particular thought or feeling we are having, how it is affecting the quality of our life, and how our situation and state of mind would change without continuing our identification with it. Very often what we discover when inquiring about our thoughts and feelings is that they are mirrors of our own inner obstructions. What we think is coming from outside is inevitably coming from inside, an interpretation being made by our identified awareness trying to protect itself. With this recognition in relation to any particular thought/feeling, the energy of the thought/feeling automatically begins to discharge. We then may choose to release the thought/feeling altogether. There are a variety of ways to release and transform thoughts and feelings. It always involves choosing in stillness, and this cultivates our sense of self beyond the body-mind.

Another style of *jnana-releasing* self-inquiry is simply allowing our awareness to be with the objects of perception – thoughts, feelings, and physical sensations – without any evaluation. As soon as we find ourselves evaluating, we just ease back to observing and allowing. In doing so, we will come to notice the endless layers of life and karmic fluctuations (causes and effects) continuously unfolding in stillness. We cannot know all of this infinite change in the mind, but we can in the infinite and timeless realm of the witness.

This sort of relationship with the objects of perception is hardly an inquiry at all, and will arise naturally over time as the witness is coming up as a result of daily deep meditation, so it is likely to begin as a form of *jnana-natural*. Then we may be inclined to make it more of an intentional practice, a voluntary letting go in the witness. It can be used not only with thoughts and feelings, but also with physical sensations that often accompany our various mental and emotional states. They are all connected. Whatever is going on with the body, mind or emotions, we can observe it in stillness, and this can bring much relief from the suffering associated with identification with the objects of perception in the body-mind. The witness has great power to dissolve obstructions in the nervous system and to release our identification with the objects of perception, simply by having the intention of allowing our increasing awareness to innocently observe. This type of releasing self-inquiry has been called *mindfulness* in the Buddhist system, and it is found in many other systems of practice as well, because it arises naturally with the witness. Gradually we develop the ability to favor that releasing mode of relationship with the objects of perception over our previously grasping and limiting identified mode.

For spiritual purposes, no system of self-inquiry is recommended to be undertaken as stand-alone. As a minimum, daily deep meditation is recommended in order to cultivate the necessary abiding inner silence. Once daily meditation is in use, *jnana-releasing* techniques can be undertaken in a measured way prior to the emergence of the abiding witness without causing undo strain. More direct forms of *jnana yoga* (affirming, negating and transcending), as discussed below, are not recommended to be approached before there is at least a beginning sense of abiding inner silence. We'd like to avoid putting excessive non-relational effort into methods of self-inquiry that look beyond the course of our ordinary daily activities. Non-relational self-inquiry can cause disruption in one's sense of wellbeing and reduce the desire to pursue a spiritual path. With prudent *self-pacing* of self-inquiry in relation to our rising inner silence (witness), such difficulties can be avoided, and the results with self-inquiry can be positive at every step along the path.

Jnana-Affirming

If we have been delving into natural self-inquiry for a while, or have been doing a structured form of *jnana-releasing* style of self-inquiry, at some point we will be looking to do more than processing the thoughts and feelings associated with ordinary everyday living. We may find ourselves looking beyond our health, our relationships, our work, our bank account and possessions, and so on. Not that these things will not matter anymore. It is only that they will be taken care of in stride, and our perspective will begin to transcend them to the more fundamental question of who we are in relation to the world from a perspective that emanates from beyond our body-mind and worldly concerns. This is caused by the continued shift of our sense of self beyond the objects of perception. At this point, we may become convinced that who we are is beyond all observed objects and phenomena. It is a revelation we can feel, and it may be interpreted by the intellect as, "I am *That.* You are *That.* All this is *That.*"

It is an ancient revelation and affirmation, dating back many centuries to the *Upanishads* and *Brahma Sutras*, and we continue to verify the profound truth of it today.

But that is only the intellect picking up on a feeling. True realization is the feeling of an expanding sense of self beyond the mind. This is not an expanding ego, though it can turn in that direction if the mind grabs on and attempts to own that feeling without sufficient ability to release it in stillness. Ego (*I, me, and mine*) is the child of mind, while the *Self* is eternal bliss consciousness. The deep-rooted mental fabrication of the ego holds on for dear life to its fragile existence in time and space, while the *Self* (in stillness) holds on to nothing and is beyond time and space. Ego mind by itself is bondage and suffering. Ego mind moving in abiding inner silence is the doorway to *liberation*.

What the mind affirms for itself is of little importance, and can become an obstruction on the path if pressed excessively at the wrong time. True affirmation is not an act of the intellect. It is an act of releasing intentions of the intellect in stillness. Intellect seeks more intellect. Affirmation seeks the *Self*, which is beyond intellect. So an affirmation is picking up an intention and letting it go. Once released, the intention of the affirmation is absorbed in stillness, where it expands in stillness as ecstatic divine flow.

The *Self* affirms nothing, even though it is everything. It is not for the mind to say. It is for the mind to surrender its impulse in stillness. Near the end of the journey, the mind can proclaim, "I am *That!*" But the words themselves are not *That*. Only when it is released in stillness can an affirmation be an aid. It can be done with any aspect of one's chosen ideal – "I am one with God," "I am one with Shiva," "I am one with Jesus," "I am *That*," etc. These are all synonymous with *Self* when released in stillness. Anything is.

This is the habit of samyama, and, as is always the case, its outcome will be according to divine flow, not necessarily our surface mental intention. The outcome of an affirmation is unfathomable. That is okay. We will get used to it. This is the way of *active surrender* to the divine flowing through us. This is the way of the *Self*. It is life in eternal love and happiness.

Jnana-Negating

Depending on our nature, we may feel inclined to take a different tact in self-inquiry. An ancient method involves *negation*, which is the systematic denial of the ego and the world as we have known it. This is the step-by-step destruction of the self-identification of awareness with all objects, including the body, thoughts, feelings, actions, and the mind itself. The premise is that awareness is eternal and that everything else is unreal, has no substance, and is to be negated. This is the mental process of inquiring on everything with the conclusion, "Not this, not this" (*neti neti*).

When we say that awareness is eternal, we do not mean that the idea of awareness is eternal, or that even the experience of awareness is eternal, for both of these are in the realm of thought and relative experience. Eternal means never born, never dies, never known. In *jnana-negating*, we become the *Self* by discarding everything else (including the idea of *Self*), just the way the emptiness of a hole is revealed by removing all the dirt in the place where the hole is.

It is like finding a beautiful statue by chipping away all the marble that is not the statue. This is the process of *neti neti*. This approach to self-inquiry was championed by none other than Adi Shankara many centuries ago, and has been revived in the public awareness in the modern era.

There is significant risk in this approach, as it is easy to get into trouble with it if undertaken as non-relational self-inquiry (not released in stillness).

<u>Negation in self-inquiry is not a negation of life.</u> If we are removing the dirt, it is presumed we will find the hole of the luminous *Self,* if we have abiding inner silence (the *witness*) to begin with, which is the luminous *Self* within us.

In that case, it may be logical and natural to drop (let go of) objects, thoughts and feelings, regarding them as unreal. However, if we don't have the witness pre-cultivated, what we may find with neti neti instead is a sense of hopelessness, fear and despair, because our sense of self will not be found in stillness yet. In that case, neti neti is not only the annihilation of our ego and the world as non-self, it is also the annihilation of our sense of self altogether with nothing there to replace it. In short, the *witness* is not easily cultivated by neti neti alone. However, the *witness* can be enlivened by neti neti if it has already been cultivated in deep meditation.

Some teachers strongly encourage the practice of *negation* early on the path, which can be psychologically (and even physically) destructive to the wellbeing of an unprepared (unripe) practitioner. When such an approach is backed with the energy of a spiritual teacher, there can be a high price to pay.

Much better to start slow and advance gradually. Rome was not built in a day.

As is the case with all practices discussed in the AYP system, *self-pacing* is recommended as necessary to maintain progress with comfort. It does not help anyone if serious overloads and dislocations occur that may take months or years to recover from. Of all the methods of self-inquiry, negation carries the greatest risk when overdoing occurs, as it can negatively impact every aspect of our life by diminishing our will to engage, which is <u>not</u> a characteristic of rising enlightenment. It is spiritual practice degenerating into an unhealthy nihilism.

So, with those cautions duly noted, the *jnana-negating* path of neti neti self-inquiry may still be attractive to some. If the negation is loving and joyful, you will know there is the resonance of inner silence there, and it can work marvelously. On the other hand, if negation is approached as a mechanical war-like process of logic, without sincere bhakti (spiritual desire), it will not work. This is true for all forms of self-inquiry. The body-mind, ego, and world are not the enemy. If we treat them as such, we will pay the price.

Jnana-Transcending

Ramana Maharshi, one of the greatest sages of the 20th century, offered a unique approach to self-inquiry that does not deal with the objects of perception at all, at least not in a common way. His enlightenment occurred outside the mainstream of traditional *jnana* and *advaita* in India, outside the guru system altogether. His approach is innovative, effective and safe. It is one of the most direct approaches to self-realization, if it is undertaken relationally, with the witness pre-cultivated in deep meditation, and with the habit of releasing intentions in stillness established (samyama).

The method is a direct inquiry into who or what the *I-sense* is. The famous question, "*Who am I?*" is at the heart of this style of self-inquiry. But first, we must notice the *I-sense*. So before we ask "*Who am I?*" we ask "*To whom is this experience right now occurring?*" The answer is obvious: It is occurring to "*I.*" Then we ask, "*Who am I?*" and let it go.

This is a process that bypasses objects of perception, because we are first asking who is experiencing them ("*I*"), and then inquire as to who or what is "*I.*" Because this approach immediately goes beyond the subject-object relationship, we call this approach *jnana-transcending*. What we realize is that the "*I*" is also an object of perception, and the inquiry as to who or what it is, takes us beyond it, transcending it.

If we look at this technique within the structure of the dynamic of observer, process of observation, and object observed, we will see that we are beginning with noticing a perception and inquiring back to the observer straight away. If our sense of self is out in the body-mind, we are still being directed back through perception to the observer. This can be easily seen with the simple inquiry, "*By whom is this body-mind being perceived?*" The answer: By "*I.*" Then we can inquire: "*Who am I?*"

Some may prefer to ask, "*What am I?*" It doesn't matter. The key to this method is identifying and inquiring on the *I-sense*, or the *I-thought*, and releasing the inquiry in stillness. It always comes back to that, and always will lead us beyond the *I-sense*.

The question, "*Who am I?*" is not to be deliberately answered in the mind. It is to be released in stillness. This is not a process of intellect. This is simple samyama that can occur as we go about our daily business.

This inquiry can also be built into our structured samyama practice by adding the sutra: "*I-thought – Who am I?*" This small addition to our twice daily samyama practice can have far-reaching long term effects in our daily life.

To the extent we use this form of self-inquiry outside our sitting practices, it should not interfere with our motivation to be active in life. If it does, we may be overdoing it, and *self-pacing* will be in order. More likely there will be a rising enthusiasm in life, coming from the effulgent *Self* we are revealing every time we release the inquiry, "*Who am I?*" relationally in stillness.

It should be emphasized that this is not a mechanical process. Asking the question "*Who am I?*" a thousand times without release in stillness will pale in its effect to doing it just once relationally (in stillness) with sincerity. Ask yourself now, what is the feeling of that question mark in "*Who am I?*" Do you really want to know who you are? If you do, and have abiding inner silence, this approach to self-inquiry can work wonders.

With *jnana-transcending*, we will sooner or later come to a deep recognition that there really is no "*I.*"

No "*me*." And no "*mine*." For what are these but fabrications of the mind via the identification of awareness with the objects of perception in the realm of time and space? The procedure of inquiring on the *I-thought* or *I-sense* eventually becomes self-contained in stillness. By then we are doing little beyond inquiring upon *stillness in stillness*, or *awareness observing awareness*. It is a natural progression from inquiring on the outer self, the *I-sense*, to inquiring on the *inner Self*, our native awareness. There is nothing beyond this, except an outpouring of *divine love* through us into all our actions in the external world. And that is pure *karma yoga*.

In going beyond the *I-sense*, we are not destroying the life we are living. We are coming into a much healthier relationship with it from the point of view of who and what we truly are – unidentified pure bliss consciousness, fully engaged and active in this world, but also not of this world. We finally come to reside in stillness in all that we do. We become *stillness in action*.

There is great power and freedom in this. But we can never own it as "*I*." To live in freedom, we must die to our identification with the objects of perception. The methods of yoga are ultimately for that, with the various approaches of *jnana yoga* being for end stage realization in stillness.

Direct Pointing – An Ancient and Modern Tool

Another angle on the *jnana-transcending* approach, which can include elements of all the other styles of *jnana yoga*, is the *direct pointing* method.

What is direct pointing?

It is first an intellectual recognition that our sense of "*I*" or the "*ego*" is an invention that has no reality of its own, except the one we have given it and habitually continue to give it. By directly observing and inquiring on the location of the "*I*," we come to the realization that it does not exist as a real thing. Such an approach can bring an immediate realization of truth, an *Aha*, if not a lasting realization. For it does not remove the need for long term purification and opening and a gradual internal neurobiological transformation leading to permanent clear seeing of the nature of reality and our *unity* with it. Enlightenment is not a state of mind, but a state of our entire neurobiological functioning, down to the last cell that sings in the divine flow. But *direct pointing* can be helpful to glimpse the truth briefly. It is an inspiration and helps awaken us. Then, what we do in practices after the initial glimpse will make all the difference.

Along these lines, it can be helpful to look further into the nature of the *I-thought* or *I-sense*. It is no different than anything else we might give a name, including our own name (John, Mary, etc.). If we call a large living plant a "tree," this does not change the reality of the tree. It is still a process of nature, doing what it does: living, growing, reproducing, etc. But naming it does change our relationship with it via the symbol we have assigned to it, overlaid upon it. On a subtle level, calling a tree a tree removes us from what the tree really is. In the world of human thought, the name designations we give everything make them separate from us. This sense of separation leads to many of the inharmonious behaviors humans have exhibited in relation to the natural environment.

It is the same with our individual names, which we know can be changed without changing the person. The objectification of human beings or groups of human beings that occurs in naming persons, ethnic groups, nations, etc., has much to do with the many conflicts we find occurring constantly in the world.

When we bring it down to the self-awareness of the individual, the first name that we recognize is "*I*." This too is a name, an objectification of a variety of sensory, mental and emotional experiences. We have called this body-mind "*I*." It separates us from the reality of what we are, just as naming a tree, or anything, separates us from the reality of that aspect of nature.

The truth of the matter is that all names are mental constructs – symbols designating processes occurring in nature, whether it is a supposedly inanimate thing (like a stone), a plant, an animal, a human being, or this body-mind we find ourselves experiencing the world through. These mental constructs are deeply embedded in our language, culture, and especially in our perception of self. Self is the deepest of all mental constructs. When that one is seen and deeply known for what it is, and for what it is not, then all the rest of the mental constructs are dissolved in the clarity of enlightened vision. This is why enlightened people are sometimes called *seers*. They see the world as it is – a living expression of unified divine flow that is continually being reinterpreted in the endless conjured up dream of human mental projection and identification.

Does this mean we should not name things, or use the concept of "*I*?" No, it doesn't mean that. The mental constructs have a purpose, of course. They enable us to function in the world. But they also are separating and limiting, and blind us to the truth of life. When we become aware of that, it is liberating, even as we continue to function using the constructs that enable us to do so with language, thinking and meaning. There is no doubt that our sense of separation from nature, which begins with identification with the *I-sense*, constitutes bondage, and is the cause of all of our suffering. But so too is our *I-sense* (ego) and our conceptual knowledge the vehicle we can ride to freedom. We can pull ourselves up by the bootstraps that way, and arrive as fully functioning liberated beings in this realm.

The methods of yoga ultimately bring us to forms of self-inquiry we have been discussing here.

In the case of "*I, me, and mine*," direct pointing is about going beyond the belief that there is really something called "*I*" in our life. There is a concept, but is there a real "*I*?"

Many things are going on: The body is moving, the mind is thinking, the emotions are moving. But is "*I*" doing anything? Is there an "*I*" doing anything at all? Direct pointing asks us to find the "*I*" that is doing anything. "*Where is the 'I' that is doing what I am doing right now?*" This is the fundamental inquiry. It is similar to identifying the *I-sense*, or *I-thought*, and then asking, "*Who or what is I?*" The answer is that there is no "*I*." It is nowhere to be found. Realizing that, then we are left as unidentified awareness observing the process of nature without the separation created by concepts, beginning with the deeply rooted concept of *"I."*

With *direct pointing* we may find overlap into other forms of inquiry to aid in seeing what is true beyond our sense of *"I."*

It may come to us naturally as a natural revelation: "Oh, there is no '*I*' here doing any of this."

The witness will gradually lead us to this revelation, and for a few, it may be all that is necessary. That is *jnana-natural*. We may take a more structured approach, using the methods of *jnana-releasing* to question the truth of our thoughts, including the many manifestations of *"I."* Is this *I-sense* true? Doesn't life go on without the *I-sense*? Yes, it does, and even better, with less suffering and more clarity and joy amidst the ups and downs of life. That is the truth. This is also an *affirmation*, which is another way of approaching direct pointing. We can also use *jnana-negating*, recognizing that there is no "*I*" at all. It has been a figment of our imagination all along. *Neti neti...*

If we do not resonate with any of these angles, it is all right. When we come to *relational self-inquiry* and *ripeness*, we will find our intuitive sense residing continually in the *witness*, which comes with the rise of abiding inner silence. A desire to cultivate that connection can be an inspiration to engage in daily deep meditation. When we do come to self-inquiry, it will be on our own terms, whether it be natural, releasing, affirming, negating, transcending, pointing, or whatever, it will be our own way, and our own awakening.

From all of this, you can see that it would not be helpful if we took a singular approach or technique from *jnana yoga* or *advaita-vedanta,* and presented it as the *AYP way.* For many yoga practices, we have been very specific, based on known causes and effects. In the case of evolution of the witness and the methods for traveling the end stage of the journey, success will come much more according to individual inclinations. That is why you find a broad survey of self-inquiry methods here. It is up to you to find what resonates for you and move ahead whenever you are ready, in *ripeness*, of course. For each practitioner, it will be a little different.

A lot is at stake in this – the quality of our daily life, going through its many ups and downs, and being able to help ourselves and others in a condition of permanent freedom.

In the ancient knowledge of the East, human bondage through identification with the *I-sense* has been called the *mistake of the mind*. But can we blame the mind? It is the nature of awareness to become identified with nature, invent objects in the mind, and interact with them in a self-created realm of illusion, or *Maya,* as it is called in Sanskrit. It has been likened to a *dream state*, a kind of ongoing *hypnosis*. And enlightenment is simply *waking up*.

But, as we have been discussing, waking up is not quite as simple as waking up in the morning. The truth is, it is intention in the heart expressed via the mind, along with the physical and all other aspects of our nature, that enable us to gradually unravel our identification with the *I-sense* and wake up.

Whatever the cause, there need be no blame. We can all agree that identification of awareness with the *I-sense* (mistaking it for self) is the culprit, and the methods of yoga provide a clear and logical way beyond that bondage, that dream state.

From the ancient *Astavakra Gita (VIII.4)*, we read:

"When there is no 'I', there is liberation.
When there is 'I', there is bondage.
Considering thus, easily refrain
from accepting or rejecting anything."

So this knowledge has been around for a long time. It is very practical, once we have effective means for going beyond the identification of awareness with the objects of perception. It is only then that we can see the *I-sense* in a balanced perspective and easily refrain from "accepting or rejecting anything." And we will know what that is about in the deepest experiential sense. It is not passivity in life. It is life conducted in the freedom of *active surrender*, as we increasingly operate from a much deeper sense of *Self*.

While we may understand the concept of no "*I*" intellectually, maybe even tasting it a bit, it will take more to travel the path. It is the entire human nervous system that contains within it the tendencies and abilities for awakening to liberation. And reflecting in our actions what is already within us, it is the methods found in yoga that gradually join our inner and outer nature in the fullness of enlightenment. Yoga is an expression of our full potential longing to emerge.

Direct pointing is one aspect of that, which we come to as our ripeness for *liberation* awakens with the rise of abiding inner silence.

The Power of the Pen, and the Keyboard

No matter which style of *jnana yoga* and self-inquiry we may be inclined toward, it will be an inner process. In fact, it can be said that we all come to spiritual practices through an inner dialogue.

No doubt we heard or read somewhere about the possibilities for improving the quality of our life though deep meditation and other practical techniques. But before we did anything about it, an inner conversation occurred. A conversation with our self. Or, more accurately, a conversation with our *Self* (big "*S*") occurred, meaning an interaction within the stillness of our inner realm, the guru in us, which is always drawing us toward more fullness and happiness in life. Once we made this connection, even a little, we sensed it was time to act, and did. Through an ongoing inner dialogue we have continued with our practices over the weeks, months and years, moving steadily closer to the freedom of enlightenment.

Writing can be a great aid on our spiritual path. When we put words on a page or a screen, we are seeing a version of our inner dialogue. We call it a "version," because, depending on how many weeks, months or years we have been writing, what we see may be a clear or distorted view of our inner-most vibrations. Writing is like a mirror of our inner life. The more developed the mirror, the clearer the view. Of course, if our inner life is in shambles, we will see that in our writing too, and there we may find opportunities to help ourselves work things out, much the way we might in an inner dialogue. The advantage of writing is that we can generally see it better than the constantly shifting multitude of our thoughts, feelings and sensations. Once we have written it down, there it is, staring us back in the face. Writing can greatly simplify things. When we see our inner condition reflected on the page, what will we do with that?

This down to earth "in your face" characteristic of writing makes it good for problem-solving at any level of perception, and especially for *self-inquiry*, no matter what style we may be drawn to. But writing is about more than problem solving. As our writing becomes more reflective of our inner nature through practice, and as we advance with internal purification and opening through daily spiritual practices, then writing can take us much deeper into perceiving our inner dialogue. It can become a reflection of the most subtle vibrations within us – a reflection of our most subtle stirrings in stillness. In other words, *relational self-inquiry*.

In this, there can be levels of perception and creativity that were not available to us before, a pipeline from that place in us where great power and genius live. Through writing, we can become a channel for that. And who knows what good may come from it? It is the place in us that is eternal and knows no fear. It is the divine wellspring. Writing can put us directly in touch with *That*. There is a progression going from external, relatively random and internally uninformed writing, to an internal, highly illuminated kind of writing. If we keep up our spiritual practices, and keep writing, these two areas of development can merge in a divine outpouring.

All of this is for our growth, and ultimately for the growth of everyone. When we take our internal dialogue, by whatever written means (prose, poetry, fiction, etc.), and express it, it forms a path that we can follow. Whether we are asking ourselves questions, or stating principles of truth, right or wrong, we will be duly affected, and grow. The penetration into truth we can find in writing is undeniable. We will be changed by it.

Private journaling has long been known to be a useful self-improvement method. When combined with daily spiritual practices such as deep meditation, spinal breathing pranayama, samyama, self-inquiry, karma yoga and related techniques, our writing can take us into new dimensions that can inspire and inform us. As a minimum, regular writing can encourage us to continue our daily practices, because we can see more clearly the changes that are occurring in us, in the mirror of our steadily refining written words. That alone makes writing highly valuable.

Besides being a tool for self-communication and an aid to our individual spiritual development, writing can be a tool for sharing our inner dialogue with others, and for communicating with others for their benefit. If we write to other individuals or to the public, we will usually be doing both at the same time

– sharing our inner life for our own benefit, and helping others to come in closer contact with their own truth.

Writing is a fluid medium that springs from our shared inner source. Because of this underlying connection, sooner or later our writing will purify and become a reflection of the inner silence that we are. The same is true for all of life. Our source cannot remain hidden from us forever. The deeper we go with writing, the deeper we go into ourselves. With spiritual practices in play, our writing will eventually become a pure reflection of the expanding inner life resulting from the natural process of human spiritual transformation. And this can be shared with many. As it goes around, the power of truth can be amplified in those who are reading with a powerful resonance. There is great transforming power in this.

Individual journaling on a regular basis can be a boon to our spiritual practice, and to our inquiry into the truth of our nature. It is always good to keep in touch with the divine within us. If we can release the question in stillness, the answer will be there. In this way, writing can be an important facilitator of our liberation.

Love of the Self

Whatever our approach to human spiritual transformation may be, and to self-inquiry and end stage liberation, the character of the *witness* will steadily evolve from a flat separate awareness to a luminous flowing aliveness that we will see expressing through the nervous system and everywhere. We have called it a *divine outpouring* and *stillness in action*. Whatever we call it, we come to realize that this is not only who we are and the *Self* of all, but also that it is *unbounded love* flowing for us, through us, and for everyone.

It is impossible not to fall completely and totally in love with this *Self*. We may call it God, or by any name that resonates with our perception of the divine. It is *Self*. It is God. In one way or other, it is the object of our bhakti, and has been the essence of our chosen ideal since the beginning. The bhakti we have experienced has always been an expression of *That*. We have never been alone. And now *IT* comes before us in fullness, expressing through the vehicle of our nervous system. The experiential recognition of this is a milestone in dissolving the limited self in the eternally joyous *Self*. We have been that in seed form all along, and by our dedication and effort, we can move beyond the witness stage and realize *That* in fullness.

Dissolving the Witness in Unity

We may fall in love with our divine *Self*, and this may tie in with our religious background, or perhaps with an intuitive sense of truth within us we have carried with us since childhood. Our spiritual desire and love of truth (bhakti) will carry us forward. But, you know, even the *Self* will be transcended.

Here we are using the terms *Self*, *inner silence* and *witness* synonymously, meaning, the pure bliss consciousness we come to know ourselves to be. But the naming of *That* is only a perceptual thought, and the truth is beyond all names and perceptions. Not that there is anything wrong with perception. Certainly we do not wish to stop perceiving in this world. We would not be able to function without the mechanics of subject, object, and the machinery of perception. Neither can we function without the *I-sense*, and even some sense of *me* and *mine*. These are all aspects of an operating body-mind in the world, where we are living right now. We don't have to suspend the operations of these aspects of life to be liberated. We only have to recognize that they are part of the divine. We are not doing them. They are doing themselves as stillness moves within, through and around us. It is all us, or *unity*.

So, while the recognition of the witness as our *Self* is very useful as we approach liberation by whatever means resonates with us, at some point we will move beyond our identification with our own abiding inner silence. It will still be there, even more so, as a feature of our existence in this realm, just as all the other aspects of our nature will be. But we will no longer be identified with the witness any more than we are identified with the *I-sense*.

So then, who is left once the witness is transcended? No one. Yet, it is all going on. But who is doing it? No one. It is the mystery of *stillness in action*.

Then we find ourselves in the paradox of enlightenment, which is a fountain of peace, joy and creativity, and doing everything while we are doing nothing. We neither accept nor reject anything, yet engage with an energy of purpose that is very powerful, with harmony overflowing in all aspects of life.

When inner silence is abiding, and we no longer see ourselves to be the witness of objects, this is what it is, and we live quite normally, in absolute freedom. Not even death can overcome us. For what is death but a ceasing of the processes of identified awareness that we have already moved beyond? It is also the ceasing of noticing the witness as an object of perception. After all, the subject (us, or *That*) cannot be an object of perception, and this is the meaning of moving beyond the witness into a sense of self which can no longer be perceived as an object.

What is it then, this awareness that cannot be perceived as self, or *Self*, being beyond all perception whatsoever?

This might beg the question: Is there awareness after death? It is a source of fascination to speculate intellectually on this, but the more fundamental question would be, is there awareness before death? The question of awareness after death we can't do much with. It either is or it isn't, and we won't know experientially until we get there. But the question of awareness before death we can do a lot with, in the here and now. We can become free in this life by addressing it with effective means, and that will bring us freedom in all future lives, if any.

In liberation, life continues to go on in ordinary ways. We may well have our old thoughts, feelings, and reactions in life but they will not pull us out of liberation. Getting rid of thoughts and feelings is not a prerequisite for *unity*. But transcending our identification with them is. This is the key point.

And, yes, our conduct will be affected much for the better, but not as dramatically as might be imagined.

There are many nuances to dissolving of the witness in *unity*. All our attitudes, expectations and judgments will be swallowed up in it. That is what happens as true non-duality is stabilizing. But it is not getting rid of our thoughts or personality. It is not passive. It is not philosophical. Nor is it an absolutist view or belief. It is a direct experience.

We must participate consciously in it to advance. How do we do that? By cultivating a sincere relationship between our native awareness (the witness, our *Self*) and all that we see going on in our life, from external relationships to our deepest attitudes and feelings about ourselves and the world we perceive around us. We will know we are on the right track when we are able to question the truth of each and every thought we have, and be able to allow it without identifying with it, without buying into it. Indeed, the questioning will be automatic, instinctual, with an immediate awareness of any discordance with the divine flow. We learn the reality of *active surrender* quite naturally.

Active Surrender

Does *active surrender* mean that we become passive in life, and unable to function? Must our mind become empty of thoughts and our life devoid of effective action in the world? No, thoughts and action will always be there. We do not suppress thoughts or actions that are appropriate for the circumstances we find ourselves in. We release our identification with them, even as we are allowing them. In doing so, our thoughts and actions rise to become divine flow. This is how *karma yoga* emerges, which is spontaneous service to others without expectation of reward. Liberation is not a retreat from life in the world. It is ongoing engagement as divine flow on many levels, seen and unseen.

As discussed in the previous section, we can choose to become active in surrendering our stories and dramas (and our knee-jerk reactions) to what is happening right now, even as the stories and dramas continue to play in our head. That's fine. Let them play. We just release in stillness and live our life. In doing so, we become pure expressions of *Being* in the world.

It is impossible to do this without the abiding witness. Without it, there will be limited space to release into, and no condition of relationship with stillness in which to inquire, allow and surrender. The relationship of the witness with our thoughts, feelings, and perceptions of the external environment is the flash point where our inquiry can gain traction. We can let go. This is where the habit of samyama can help us. It all must be released. We can't own anything, not a thought, not a feeling, not even the witness itself. The thoughts and feelings will be there, the witness will be there, but we can release our ownership of them. When we can do this honestly in an inquiring way, and the habit comes to abide in us, then we find that everything is in us, and we own it all without owning anything. We are free!

Jesus said we must die to be born again in this life. This is what we do. In letting go of it all, we gain it all. It is the *divine paradox*. There can be some discomfort as this process is unfolding, a feeling that we are losing something, or losing everything. It is a natural reaction, one that we will get over as we proceed. In the end, we will find that we are still here, more than ever before, and free. Nothing will be lost but our illusions about life, and everything will be gained.

By keeping active and engaged in life, we will find that all the discomforts and expectations we have in daily living will be our intimate teachers. When we can embrace these, allowing them and interpenetrating them without clinging or judgment, then that is the dissolving of the witness in *unity*.

If we run away into the witness and do not engage in life, we will be in a trap of our own making. Do not let the tricky mind off the hook so easily. Give the mind no safe perch on which to land. It habitually will try to keep us identified outside the essence of what we are. By fearlessly noticing and dissolving what we are not, what is not true, we will become what we are, which surpasses our imagined egoic self by infinite measure.

It is a tall order, even though it is only recognizing that less is more. It is something that each of us will approach in our own way, according to our natural inclinations at any point in time.

It is not recommended to tackle this head-on prior to the dawn of the abiding witness, and not recommended beyond the point of keeping a stable lifestyle and daily practice routine. If we find ourselves struggling with self-inquiry in daily life, or are wallowing with apathy in the witness, it will be a sign of imbalance, too much on one side or the other of the edge. Then it will be time for an adjustment – either to self-pace in practices, or to get up off the couch and go out and live fully.

Going Beyond the Witness

Is going beyond the witness a state of emptiness, or void?

The witness and emptiness/void are two aspects of the same thing. The witness is awareness with objects. How could there be a witness with nothing to witness? But emptiness can be present with or without objects. So the witness is emptiness with objects.

It's the same with consciousness. We use the word all the time – pure bliss consciousness and all that – but it only has meaning when there is something to be conscious of. Consciousness is awareness being conscious through a body-mind. Beyond the body-mind, it is empty/void.

Emptiness/void is awareness with no objects. Nothing to be aware of. Pure potential, beyond all that exists. The source of all. We can also be that in the body-mind. We are *That*. It expresses as consciousness and the witness through the body-mind, and as everything we see and do.

The question arises, can awareness exist with no vehicle, no body? Is emptiness/void aware? How can we know? That is why the words emptiness and void are used.

Awareness in emptiness is left as an open question. Quantum physics is at this point in its scientific inquiry also, where everything we see is known to be nothing but energy moving in emptiness. But look around. Miracles are happening all the time, so why not eternal awareness? I'm game for it if you are. At any rate, awareness is now. We have it, and we are it. That we know. So it is suggested to take the necessary steps to live it fully in *unity* in this life. That is freedom. That is liberation, and it is available to all human beings.

Chapter 4 – Liberation

We started off this discussion exploring liberation, also called enlightenment, somewhat speculatively in terms of what it may be, and how we might progress toward it if we choose to. Most everyone has had an inkling of it in this era of spiritual awaking amidst the remaining dark shadows of our era. They say it is darkest before the dawn, but even in the darkness, there will be signs of the coming light. And we are seeing that now, with so many becoming attuned to their inner process of awaking.

Once we have had a taste of our true nature, what we do after that will make all the difference.

If we have been wise in pursuing a path of daily spiritual practice, then what was only a glimmer, a brief peak experience, can be cultivated and stabilized to transform our experience in this life entirely.

Unending peace, energy, and creativity are available to us. All we need to do is apply the time-tested methods for unfolding it. Then we come to know that freedom is not a figment of our imagination, but a reality that we can live every day, without having to retreat into a cave or run away to a mountain top. Liberation is here and now. We have no place to go but within ourselves each day, and bring the inner quality out into our daily activity.

It is very simple.

We Are That

It is one thing to say it is simple, and quite something else to take the simple steps that hasten the process of human spiritual transformation. It does take a certain amount of clarity and persistence to make the journey. It will not happen entirely by itself. There is cause and effect in all things, including on the spiritual path.

It is like the simplicity of going from New York to California these days. All we have to do is get on an airplane, and a few hours later we are there. But how simple is it to get to California if we don't get on the airplane? Can we sit in New York and will ourselves to California? Maybe if we are among the rarest of human beings we can. But everyone else will have to get on the airplane.

Yoga and the journey to liberation are like that. It is an easy path, if we take it. If we don't take it, and try to will our way to liberation instead, it can be very tough. A few might discourage us from getting on the path of doing anything, but it will not be realistic for the vast majority of us. So the first thing is to commit ourselves to the journey, and then take the necessary steps. If we do that, it is very easy.

We have covered the means in detail throughout the AYP writings. In this book, we have focused on the end stage, which is about our neurobiology reaching a stage of ripeness suitable for completing the process of transcending identification with all objects of perception. That is not an intellectual transcending, but an experiential transcending in our daily life, even when we are not thinking about it.

Liberation is not an intellectual conditioning. Not an aloof condition of mind. It is something that awakens deep within us, where we are known to be abiding inner silence, and deeply engaged in the processes of life at the same time. It is direct knowledge, without any sort of content or qualifier. That is what we are when we are realized, when we are enlightened, when we are liberated. Then we are doing as we always did, and more, but without doing. We come to know ourselves to be the essence of everything, and with great power in the world. But at the same time, we find that we are no one and nowhere.

Yet, in that no-oneness and no-whereness, we are pure bliss consciousness, constantly full to overflowing, beyond suffering, and eternally free.

We are *That*.

Stillness in Action and Outpouring Divine Love

Life in liberation is a contradiction, and perhaps that is why those who have tried to share it have had so little success in conveying it to others. The only tools we have for approaching the miracle of enlightenment are body, mind, and heart. If we use all of these with informed purpose, we will be on our way. More often than not, the mind attempts to do it alone, particularly when the vision of possibilities seems so obvious. But what is obvious to the mind, is not so obvious to the neurobiology, which requires purification and opening before it can support the kind of functioning that underlies the enlightenment experience on a full time basis.

So the journey is 90% about the prerequisites, maybe even 99% about the prerequisites – for the process of becoming *ripe*. Only then can the fruit be picked, or fall off the tree by itself. It is the tail end of a long process. If we try to start with the picking, and press with the picking, we will still have to get to the ripened stage. That is how it is.

Once we do become ripe and are falling into the enlightened stage, what we have called *unity*, then many contradictions will arise. What could be more contradictory than *stillness in action*? It is an oxymoron!

Outpouring of divine love is a bit easier for the mind to grasp. The human being becomes a channel for that. But in that, the sense of individual self is dissolving, and that may not be so easy to grasp. One cannot happen without the other. Personal needs may stand in the way of the divine flow at times. This becomes apparent as our life becomes an expression of *stillness in action*, and we learn to adapt accordingly through *active surrender*.

If we have taken the steps to become ripe, there will be no confusion about the transformation, because we will have noticed it going on by degrees for a long time. As we become stillness, our life becomes an expression of stillness. As our intentions and inquiries are automatically released in stillness, then whatever comes out from that will be divine flow. As this way of living becomes natural to us, it increases to become an outpouring. That is how it comes to us, as a natural evolution of the cause and effect of daily practices, and our engagement in the world as a blend of inner silence (stillness) and ecstatic conductivity (energy/action). The process of living fully merges these two qualities of our divine nature deep within us, and all the way out into every aspect of our daily life. Then we come to know life as the marriage of stillness and action. We are living the paradox, and it makes perfect sense.

Freedom

"Freedom." What does it mean? Is it worth having? How do we get it? These are relevant questions. Perhaps the most relevant of our life.

We live in an age where many enjoy political and economic freedom. Hopefully human civilization will continue to evolve in a direction that brings that kind of freedom to everyone on the earth.

But we are not talking about that kind of freedom here. We are talking about a kind of freedom that transcends political and economic circumstances, a kind of freedom that transcends the suffering found in all the circumstances of life, whether we are happy, sad, rich, poor, healthy or sick. We'd all like to better our lot in life. But beyond that, there is a way to find an inner unending joy that is entirely independent of our lot in life, whatever it may be. This is what we mean by *freedom* in the yogic sense. True freedom is the fruition of yoga. It has also been called *liberation*.

This freedom, this liberation, is not an external thing, and not an idea or a state of mind. It is not something we can possess. It is a condition of consciousness in the human being, and is also reflected in the consciousness of the society. It is something that is self-evident when it appears, and entirely independent of our outer circumstances. It is an abiding inner silence, a blissful ecstasy, and an endless outpouring of divine love. Most importantly, it is freedom from suffering. It is also a direct experience of *Oneness* (unity) through all the faculties of perception. It is living within and through the essence of what we are – pure bliss consciousness. Human beings are designed to express that reality in the realm of time and space, and in ordinary daily living.

If we wait long enough, evolution will bring the human race to a full expression of that condition of freedom. Without our direct participation, it could take a very long time. But, thankfully, that is not how the system works. There is something in us, something that causes us to take action for the benefit of our evolution in this life. Once we have sensed our potential, there is a spark of recognition, and we are moved to do something. We experience a divine desire for that which is beyond where we are today in the expression of our consciousness. We have called that desire "*bhakti*," which is devotion to a higher ideal of our own choosing. There are a variety of experiences that can create that spark of recognition and the resulting bhakti. Once it happens, we have to do something. There is no turning back. We are on the path to freedom.

There are many ways to travel. We can take a religious route or a non-religious route. Whatever suits our nature. All routes lead to the same place, to the extent they are true to the inner dynamics of human spiritual transformation. In spite of all the glitz and glamour, spiritual development is largely a mechanical process. A pretty mundane thing. It is inner purification and opening of our nervous system at the deepest level that ultimately brings about freedom. A systematic approach involving daily practice will yield the most reliable results.

In the AYP system of practices, two primary angles of approach are recognized and addressed, leading to a third, which is the unfoldment of freedom.

- The cultivation of abiding blissful inner silence.

- The cultivation of ecstatic conductivity and radiance.

- The joining of these two in an outpouring of ecstatic bliss and *unity* in daily living.

One, two, three… Very simple.

To enable this process to occur, an arsenal of tools has been presented throughout the AYP writings, beginning with the core practices of deep meditation and spinal breathing pranayama, and with many additional practices and variations on practices available to facilitate the three-step process in as flexible a manner as may be needed.

It is our own direct experience that will drive our actions on the path. We can have the greatest blessings of the sages, and all the tools in the world, but if we are not willing to take responsibility for our development, driven by our direct experiences, our journey will be out of balance, out of kilter, and not very progressive. Taking personal responsibility is the key on our path to freedom. Isn't this the case with anything that is important to us?

The AYP system is designed for those who have realized this and are interested in proceeding in a self-directed manner. No one else can do it for us. The resources on practices are openly available and plentiful, the community support is considerable, and the guidelines on *self-pacing* of practices to facilitate progressive and stable inner purification and opening have been tested by thousands who have gone before. It is an approach that works. Many are advancing along their path according to their own efforts in twice-daily practice.

But there is something more. We have called it "*getting ripe*" and falling off the tree of duality into the non-dual condition, which is *unity*. This is the province of *self-inquiry*, which has been expanded upon in this volume. While we can find great joy and excitement at every step along the path, ultimate freedom is found in realizing the non-dual condition of *unity*. It is here that we know ourselves to be fully in but not of this world, and no longer susceptible to the suffering associated with the identification of awareness with the body, mind, emotions, and sensory perceptions. This is not primarily a state of mind or an intellectual understanding. We simply find that we are not any of these things, and that we are all of them. It is a mystery.

Freedom is an unknowing in which all is known. In that knowing, all can be accomplished without limit. The process of getting ripe for this is primarily about the cultivation of abiding inner silence, stillness, which we have also called the witness. The rise of ecstatic conductivity and radiance also has a key role in enabling stillness (witness) to move outward. With the rise of the witness, we find a separation of our sense of self from the objects of perception, including thoughts, feelings, sensory perceptions, and also our sense of "*I, me, and mine.*" In stillness/witness and with inquiries released in stillness, we "go out" beyond identified awareness – the attachment that leads to suffering. But this is only half of it. This is a dual condition of unidentified awareness (witness), with everything else being an object – it is still subject and objects. The other half is a "coming back" into relationship with all the objects, including our sense of "*I,*" with a merging in stillness. Then there is no longer subject (awareness) and objects, but a *unity* of subject and objects. This is *Oneness*, the freedom that is the fruition of yoga.

First it is about becoming ripe, primarily with sitting practices, and other considerations in our daily living and lifestyle. Once we are becoming ripe, having increasing abiding inner silence, then there is a role for self-inquiry. Finally, when we have gone out beyond identification with objects and come back into the *unity* of merged subject and objects, we are free, and continue to help others as we are naturally inclined, moving from within in a natural divine flow.

The journey to freedom is not an overnight affair. It is a marathon, not a sprint. But it is a much shorter marathon than it has been in the past. World consciousness has become considerably more fluid than in the past. More can be accomplished with spiritual practices these days than at any time in our known history. And there are many more options for practice available. So it is a pretty good situation. Still, there is much to do.

The AYP writings are a resource. Certainly not the only approach available, but one that is effective and open to all. There are no limits or requirements for the use of AYP, except for each of us to endeavor to be true to our own journey. It is suggested to aim for the long term in daily practice, while taking it one day at a time. In the now, but not caught up in the now. Do your best to release expectations as much as possible (difficult sometimes), always gently favoring the procedures of practice over the many experiences that will come up along the way. This is the surest path forward.

With this straight-forward approach, stillness will rise and begin to move in blissfully ecstatic ways in daily living, carrying us forward like water running downhill. No obstacle can stand in the way of the awakened divine flow. Let go in the flow, and you will realize that you are the flow, a marriage of human and divine. This is freedom.

Share with others as you are so inclined, so many can move onward into freedom, wherever they may be.

I wish you all the best on your path. It is in your hands.

The guru is in you.

Further Reading and Support

Yogani is an American spiritual scientist who, for forty years, has been integrating ancient techniques from around the world which cultivate human spiritual transformation. The approach is non-sectarian, and open to all. His books include:

Advanced Yoga Practices – Easy Lessons for Ecstatic Living (Two Volumes)
Two large user-friendly textbooks providing over 400 detailed lessons on the AYP integrated system of practices.

The Secrets of Wilder – A Novel
The story of young Americans discovering and utilizing actual secret practices leading to human spiritual transformation.

The AYP Enlightenment Series
Easy-to-read instruction books on yoga practices, including:

- *Deep Meditation – Pathway to Personal Freedom*
- *Spinal Breathing Pranayama – Journey to Inner Space*
- *Tantra – Discovering the Power of Pre-Orgasmic Sex*
- *Asanas, Mudras and Bandhas – Awakening Ecstatic Kundalini*
- *Samyama – Cultivating Stillness in Action, Siddhis and Miracles*
- *Diet, Shatkarmas and Amaroli – Yogic Nutrition and Cleansing for Health and Spirit*
- *Self-Inquiry – Dawn of the Witness and the End of Suffering*
- *Bhakti and Karma Yoga – The Science of Devotion and Liberation Through Action*
- *Eight Limbs of Yoga – The Structure and Pacing of Self-Directed Spiritual Practice*
- *Retreats – Fast Track to Freedom – A Guide for Leaders and Practitioners*
- *Liberation – The Fruition of Yoga*

For up-to-date information on the writings of Yogani, and for the free *AYP Support Forums*, please visit:

www.advancedyogapractices.com

www.ingramcontent.com/pod-product-compliance
Lightning Source LLC
Chambersburg PA
CBHW020006290326

41935CB00007B/322